RAPID NURSING INTERVENTIONS:

Respiratory

Delmar Publishers' Online Services
To access Delmar on the World Wide Web, point your browser to:
http://www.delmar.com/delmar.html
To access through Gopher:
gopher://gopher.delmar.com
(Delmar Online is part of "thomson.com," an Internet site with information on more than 30 publishers of the International Thomson Publishing organization.)
For more information on our products and services:
email: info@delmar.com or call 800-347-7707

RAPID NURSING INTERVENTIONS:

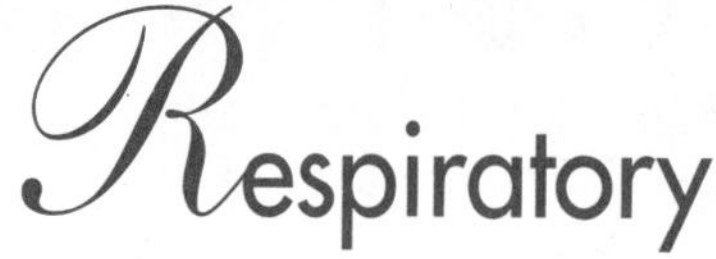

Mark B. Bauman, RN, BSN, CCRN
Full Partner, Neurotrauma ICU
R. Adams Cowley Shock Trauma Center
University of Maryland Medical Center
Baltimore

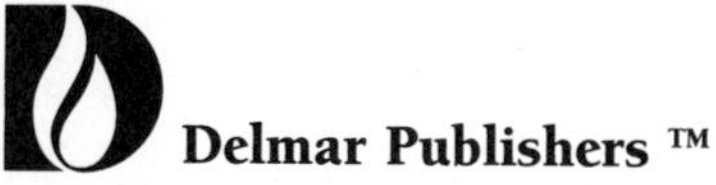

I(T)P™ An International Thomson Publishing Company

Albany • Bonn • Boston • Cincinnati • Detroit • London • Madrid
Melbourne • Mexico City • New York • Pacific Grove • Paris • San Francisco
Singapore • Tokyo • Toronto • Washington

STAFF

Team Leader:
DIANE McOSCAR

Sponsoring Editors:
PATRICIA CASEY
BILL BURGOWER

Developed for Delmar Publishers by:
JENNINGS & KEEFE Media Development, Corte Madera, CA

Concept, Editorial, and Design Management:
THE WILLIAMS COMPANY, LTD., Collegeville, PA

Project Coordinator:
KATHLEEN LUCZAK

Editorial Administrator:
GABRIEL DAVIS

Production Editor:
BARBARA HODGSON

Manuscript written by:
TERRI A. GREENBERG

Research Assistant:
MONIKA BAUMAN, RN, BSN, CEN

Text Design:
KM DESIGN GROUP

For information, address:
Delmar Publishers
3 Columbia Circle
Box 15015
Albany, NY 12212-5015

International Thomson Publishing Europe
Berkshire House 168-173
High Holborn
London, WC1V7AA
England

Thomas Nelson Australia
102 Dodds Street
South Melbourne, 3205
Victoria, Australia

Nelson Canada
1120 Birchmount Road
Scarborough, Ontario
Canada M1K 5G4

International Thomson Editores
Campos Eliseos 385, Piso 7
Col Polanco
11560 Mexico D F Mexico

International Thomson Publishing GmbH
Königswinterer Strasse 418
53227 Bonn
Germany

International Thomson Publishing Asia
221 Henderson Road
#05-10 Henderson Building
Singapore 0315

International Thomson Publishing Japan
Hirakawacho Kyowa Building, 3F
2-2-1 Hirakawacho
Chiyoda-ku, Tokyo 102
Japan

Printed in the United States of America

Published simultaneously in Canada by Nelson Canada, a division of The Thomson Corporation.

1 2 3 4 5 6 7 8 9 10 XXX 00 99 98 97 96 95

Library of Congress Cataloging-in-Publication Data
Bauman, Mark B., 1963-
Rapid nursing interventions: respiratory/Mark B. Bauman
p. cm. — (Rapid nursing interventions)
Includes bibliographical references and index.
ISBN 0-8273-7095-4
1. Respiratory organs—Diseases—Nursing. I. Title.
II. Series.
[DNLM: 1. Respiratory Tract Diseases—nursing—handbooks. 2. Respiratory Tract Diseases—diagnosis—nurses' instruction—handbooks. 3. Nursing Diagnosis—handbooks. WY 49 B3469r 1995]
RC735.5.838 1995
610.73'692—dc20
DNLM/DLC
for Library of Congress 95-23167
CIP

TITLES IN THIS SERIES:

INSTANT NURSING ASSESSMENT:

- ▲ Cardiovascular
- ▲ Respiratory
- ▲ Neurologic
- ▲ Women's Health
- ▲ Gerontologic
- ▲ Mental Health
- ▲ Pediatric

RAPID NURSING INTERVENTIONS:

- ▲ Cardiovascular
- ▲ Respiratory
- ▲ Neurologic
- ▲ Women's Health
- ▲ Gerontologic
- ▲ Mental Health
- ▲ Pediatric

Series Advisor:
Helene K. Nawrocki, RN, MSN, CNA
Executive Vice President
The Center for Nursing Excellence
Newtown, Pennsylvania
Adjunct Faculty, La Salle University
Philadelphia, Pennsylvania

Series Review Board
Irma D'Antonio, RN, Ph.D.
Associate Professor and Chairperson,
Department of Family Nursing
College of Nursing
University of North Carolina
Charlotte, North Carolina

Mary A. Baroni, RN, Ph.D.
Assistant Professor,
School of Nursing
University of Wisconsin-Madison
Madison, Wisconsin

Katherine G. Bowman, RN, MS(N)
Instructor and Co-Coordinator,
Nursing of Women & Newborns
University of Missouri at Columbia
Columbia, Missouri

Noreen Esposito, Ed.D., WHNP
Assistant Professor of Nursing
University of South Florida
Tampa, Florida

Cynthia Lynne Fenske, RN, MS
Lecturer, School of Nursing
Acute, Critical, and Long-Term Care
University of Michigan
Ann Arbor, Michigan

Diane Schwede Jedlicka, RN, CCRN, MS
Associate Professor, Nursing Department
Otterbein College
Westerville, Ohio

Sandra J. MacKay, RN, Ph.D.
Professor, Department of Nursing
San Francisco State University School of Nursing
San Francisco, California

Suzanne K. Marnocha, RN, MSN, CCRN
Assistant Professor, College of Nursing
University of Wisconsin
Oshkosh, Wisconsin

Linda Moody, RN, FAAN, Ph.D.
Professor, Director of Research and Chair,
Gerontology Nursing, College of Nursing
University of South Florida
Tampa, Florida

Patricia A. O'Neill, RN, CCRN, MSN
Instructor, DeAnza College School of Nursing
Cupertino, California

Virgil Parsons, RN, DNSc, Ph.D.
Professor, School of Nursing
San Jose State University
San Jose, California

Elaine Rooney, MSN
Assistant Professor of Nursing, Nursing Department
University of Pittsburgh
Bradford, Pennsylvania

Barbara Shafner, RN, Ph.D.
Associate Professor, Department of Nursing
Otterbein College
Westerville, Ohio

Elaine Souder, RN, Ph.D.
Associate Professor, College of Nursing
University of Arkansas for Medical Sciences
Little Rock, Arkansas

Mary Tittle, RN, Ph.D.
Associate Professor, College of Nursing
University of South Florida
Tampa, Florida

Peggy L. Wros, RN, Ph.D.
Assistant Professor of Nursing
Linfield College School of Nursing
Portland, Oregon

CONTENTS

NOTICE TO THE READER

The publisher, editors, advisors, and reviewers do not warrant or guarantee any of the products described herein nor have they performed any independent analysis in connection with any of the product information contained herein. The publisher, editors, advisors, and reviewers do not assume, and each expressly disclaims, any obligation to obtain and include information other than that provided to them by the manufacturer.

The reader is expressly warned to consider and adopt all safety precautions that might be indicated by the activities described herein and to avoid all potential hazards. By following the instructions contained herein, the reader willingly assumes all risks in connection with such instructions.

The publisher, editors, advisors, and reviewers make no representations or warranties of any kind, including but not limited to the warranties of fitness for particular purpose or merchantability, nor are any such representations implied with respect to the material set forth herein, and the publisher, editors, advisors, and reviewers take no responsibility with respect to such material. The publisher, editors, advisors, and reviewers shall not be liable for any special, consequential, or exemplary damages resulting, in whole or in part, from readers' use of, or reliance upon, this material.

A conscientious effort has been made to ensure that the drug information and recommended dosages in this book are accurate and in accord with accepted standards at the time of publication. However, pharmacology is a rapidly changing science, so readers are advised, before administering any drug, to check the package insert provided by the manufacturer for the recommended dose, for contraindications for administration, and for added warnings and precautions. This recommendation is especially important for new, infrequently used, or highly toxic drugs.

CPR standards are subject to frequent change due to ongoing research. The American Heart Association can verify changing CPR standards when applicable. Recommended Schedules for Immunization are also subject to frequent change. The American Academy of Pediatrics, Committee on Infectious Diseases can verify changing recommendations.

FOREWORD

As quality and cost effectiveness continue to drive rapid change within the health-care system, you must respond quickly and surely—whether you are a student, novice, or expert. This Rapid Nursing Interventions series—and its companion Instant Nursing Assessment series—will help you do that by providing a great deal of nursing information in short, easy-to-read columns, charts and boxes. This quick, convenient presentation will support you as you practice your science and art and apply the nursing process. I hope you'll come to look on these books as providing "an experienced nurse in your pocket."

The Rapid Nursing Interventions series is a handy source for step-by-step nursing actions to meet the fast-paced challenges of today's nursing profession. The Instant Nursing Assessment series offers immediate, relevant clinical information on the most important aspects of patient assessment. These books contain several helpful special features, including nurse alerts to warn you quickly about critical assessment findings, nursing diagnoses, charts that include interventions and rationales, along with collaborative management to help you work with your health-care colleagues, patient teaching tips, and the latest nursing research findings.

Each title in the Rapid Nursing Interventions series begins with a quick review of symptoms and focused assessment followed by the components of nursing intervention. From there, each book expands to cover the essential nursing interventions and rationales, collaborative management, outcomes, and evaluation criteria for important diagnoses covered in that title.

Both medical and nursing diagnoses are included to help you adapt to emerging critical pathways, care mapping, and decision trees. All these new guidelines help decrease length-of-stay and increase quality of care—all current health-care imperatives.

I'm confident that each small but powerful volume will prove indispensable in your nursing practice. Each book is formatted to help you quickly connect your assessment findings with the patient's pathophysiology—a cognitive connection that will further help you plan nursing interventions, both independent and collaborative, to care for your patients skillfully and completely. With the help and guidance provided by the books in this series, you will be able to thrive—and survive—in these changing times.

—Helene K. Nawrocki, RN, MSN, CNA
Executive Vice President
The Center for Nursing Excellence
Newtown, Pennsylvania
Adjunct Faculty, La Salle University
Philadelphia, Pennsylvania

SECTION I. SYMPTOMS AND INTERVENTION REVIEW

Chapter 1. Symptoms and Focused Assessment

▽ ▽ ▽ ▽ ▽ ▽ ▽

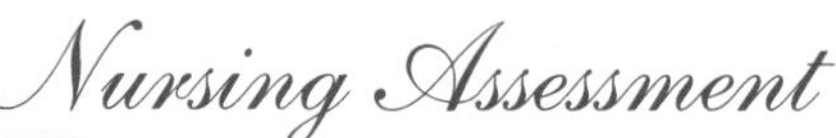

Nursing Assessment

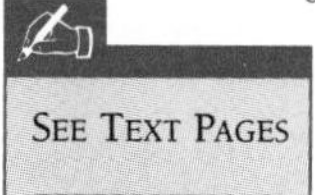

Nursing assessment is the systematic, ongoing collection, verification, and communication of data about a particular patient from various sources throughout the care of the patient. It establishes a data base of information about a patient's level of wellness, health practices, past illnesses, and health care goals and needs.

Nursing assessment is the first step of the nursing process and influences the remaining steps: diagnosis, planning, implementation, and evaluation. The information collected during assessment provides the basis of an individualized plan of care for each patient.

Two types of data are collected during nursing assessment: subjective and objective.

- Subjective data, or symptoms, are the patient's perceptions about his or her health problems. Only the patient can provide this information. It usually includes feelings of anxiety, physical discomfort, and mental distress.
- Objective data, or signs, are the observations, perceptions, and measurements made by the nurse or other data collector. This information is usually obtained through physical examination, psychosocial assessment, clinical observations, and diagnostic studies.

Included in a patient's data base are the health history, physical assessment, psychosocial assessment, review of clinical records, and review of the literature.

Health History

The following information is included in the patient's health history.

- Biographic information—factual demographic data about the patient. Age, address, working status, marital status, and types of insurance are all important types of biographic information.
- Reasons for seeking health care—expressed and recorded in the patient's own words.
- Present illness or health concern—onset (sudden or gradual), duration, location, intensity, and quality of symptoms. Precipitating and alleviating factors also need to be assessed. It is appropriate to discuss the patient's and family's expectations of the health care team so that mutual and realistic goals can be established.
- Past health history—previous hospitalizations and surgeries; allergies to food, drugs, and pollutants, with specific reactions; alcohol, tobacco, caffeine, and drug use, including frequency and duration of use; nutritional habits; previous blood transfusions; and prescribed and self-prescribed medications.
- Family history—determination of risk factors for cancer, heart disease, diabetes mellitus, kidney disease, hypertension, and mental disorders. If any of the patient's immediate blood relatives have a history of a serious disease or are being treated for such a disease, details about the disease or condition, treatment, and response should be noted in the patient's record.
- Environmental history—exposure to pollutants and threats to physical safety.
- Psychosocial and cultural history—primary language, ethnic group, affect, coping skills, spiritual and social affiliations, and developmental stage.
- Review of systems—systematic approach to obtaining information about all body systems by questioning the patient about the normal functioning of each body system. Abnormalities are clearly and concisely documented.
- Self-care abilities—ability to bathe, feed, dress, and toilet himself or herself as well as ability to walk and potentially use walking aids (cane or walker).
- Discharge planning factors—destination after discharge; support systems, including family, friends, and community resources; and access to transportation, shopping, and health care facilities.

Physical Assessment

During a physical assessment, objective data are collected to verify or negate abnormalities, identify patient needs, and appropriately establish a plan of care.

The following are important things to remember when performing a physical assessment.

- Make clear, concise explanations to the patient about what you are doing, why you are doing it, and how long the examination will take.
- Assess what is appropriate for the patient's condition; establish priorities. For example, an elderly patient who fatigues easily may require minimal position changes, and a patient with chest pain may require only a quick cardiovascular assessment rather than a neurologic examination.
- Ensure the patient's privacy and provide good lighting and a quiet, restful environment.
- Carry out a systematic, thorough physical assessment to prevent omissions in data collection. The following are two examples of physical examination methods:
  - Head-to-toe approach—systematic assessment of the patient beginning at the head and ending at the toes
  - Body systems approach—systematic assessment of the patient according to a designated sequence of body systems
- Before proceeding with the examination, the nurse should make a general survey, which includes observation information related to mental status, body development, nutritional status, sex, race, chronologic versus apparent age, appearance, and speech.

The techniques used to perform a physical assessment include the following:

- Inspection—visualizing the patient's body. Visual inspection is combined with hearing and smelling. Inspection is often the best way to begin an examination because it is the assessment technique that is least threatening to the patient.
- Palpation—examining the surface of the body with light touch using the hands or fingers and examining the deeper body structures with deep palpation. This technique may be used to evaluate organ position, body temperature, abnormal growths, and abdominal rigidity as well as to identify the location of pain.
- Percussion—sharp tapping of the body surface to produce vibration of the underlying structures. This

technique is used to determine the position and size of organs and to check for the presence of fluid or air in a body cavity.
- Auscultation—listening with a stethoscope for heart, lung, and bowel sounds.

Technique for Applying Indirect Percussion

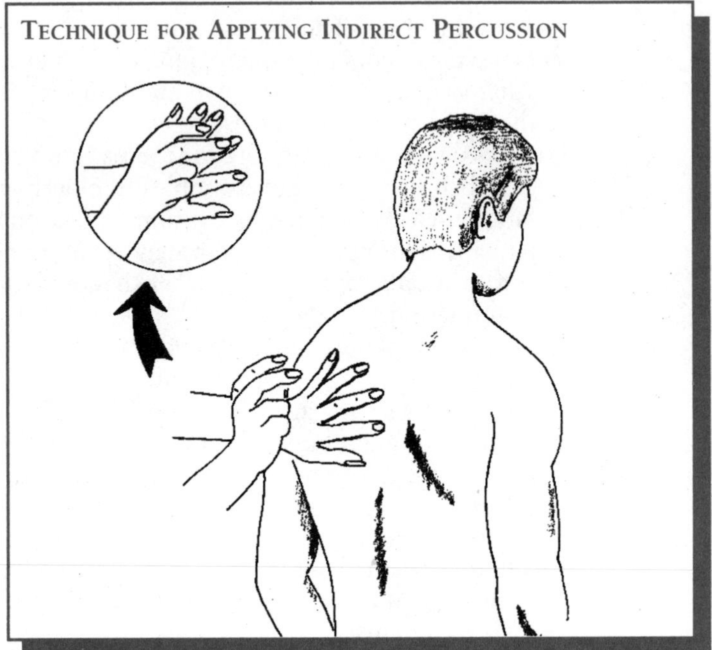

Psychosocial Assessment

- General appearance and behavior: includes motor ability, language ability, writing ability, and sensory function
- Sensorium: includes level of consciousness, orientation, attention span, memory, cognitive abilities, general knowledge, intellectual level, emotional state, and life situation
- Mental dysfunction, if present

Laboratory and Diagnostic Findings

Included in this data base component are baseline information, response to illness, and the effects of treatment methods.

The following are sources of data:

- *Interview with the patient.* The patient can usually provide the most accurate information regarding his or her health care needs, lifestyle patterns, past and present illnesses, and changes in activities of daily living. The patient interview requires effective communication techniques, including interviewing skills and active listening. The nurse needs to be calm, unhurried, and relaxed. Ideally, the environment should be quiet and free from interruptions. To conclude the interview, the nurse should summarize the main points. The patient then has the opportunity to agree or disagree with the nurse's perceptions of his or her health problems.

- *Interview with the family.* Family members can be interviewed as primary sources of information when the patient is an infant or a child or is mentally handicapped, disoriented, or unconscious. The same techniques described for a patient interview apply to a family interview.
- *Consultation with other health care professionals.* This may include physicians, physical therapists, social workers, community health workers, and clergy. These people can provide information about how the patient interacts with the health care environment, reacts to results of diagnostic procedures, and responds to visitors. This consultation may also help the nurse to gather data about the social supports that are in place in the community so that effective discharge planning can be done.

Review of Clinical Records

This review verifies information about past health patterns and treatments or provides new information.

Review of the Literature

This review completes the data base by increasing the nurse's knowledge of appropriate treatments, symptoms, prognosis, and standards of therapeutic practice.

The last part of the assessment consists of the following processes:

- Validation of data by comparison with other sources, such as a comparison of subjective data with objective data
- Organization of information into meaningful clusters with focus on areas that need support and assistance for recovery

- Documentation of data, consisting of the recording of all observations collected during assessment. The documentation should be descriptive and concise and should not include the nurse's interpretations. The origins of descriptive data are in the patient's perception of the symptoms, the family's observations, the nurse's observations, and reports from other members of the health care team.

For example, a patient may describe chest pain as "an elephant sitting on my chest." The nurse's observations may be stated as follows:

"The patient clutches his chest with both hands. Patient keeps eyes tightly closed throughout assessment."

The nurse should not interpret the patient's behavior as "the patient tolerates pain poorly."

The nurse should report the information concisely, using correct medical terminology. For example, "Patient complains of substernal chest pressure radiating to the left arm, which began 2 hours ago related to moving the left arm. The pain has not been relieved with nitroglycerin, antacids, or rest."

From the recorded data, the nurse can formulate the appropriate nursing diagnoses.

Chapter 2. Nursing Interventions

▽ ▽ ▽ ▽ ▽ ▽ ▽

Outcome Development

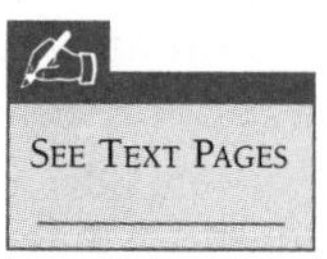

Outcomes are descriptions of the behavior that a person will display if the care plan has been successful. They demonstrate resolution or reduction of the patient's problems as presented in the nursing diagnoses. Outcome statements need to be clear, concise, realistic, and patient-centered.

Nursing Interventions

Nursing interventions are actions directed toward assisting a patient to cope successfully with physical and emotional problems and to achieve the desired outcome. There are two types of nursing interventions: independent and collaborative.

- Independent interventions are treatments a nurse can prescribe and carry out without a physician's order. They do not require collaboration with other health care professionals. Assistance with activities of daily living (ADLs) related to hygiene is an independent nursing intervention. The scope of practice that a nurse can perform independently is licensed and mandated by the nurse practice act in the state in which the nurse works. Nurse practice acts vary from state to state.
- Collaborative interventions are shared with other health care team members. Many nursing interventions require an order from a physician. The nurse's role is to carry out the order and then assess the patient for desired or unfavorable outcomes. The nurse collaborates not only with the physician but also with other members of the health care team, such as dietitians, occupational therapists, physical therapists, dance therapists, music therapists, play therapists, and social workers.

Skills

To implement interventions, the nurse needs to demonstrate cognitive skills, interpersonal skills, and technical or psychomotor skills.

- Cognitive skills are the nurse's intellectual skills, such as problem solving, decision making, critical thinking, and innovation. The nurse needs to know the rationale for each intervention and to identify patient education and discharge needs. Cognitive skills are based on the nurse's education and experience. The nurse is responsible for the development of these cognitive skills through formal and informal educational opportunities.
- Interpersonal skills are the verbal and nonverbal communication skills that are used with the patient, family members, and health care team. The nurse must be able to communicate a concerned and caring attitude and to teach and counsel at a level compatible with the patient's understanding and emotional response.
- Technical or psychomotor skills are those used during implementation—for example, to prepare an injection, change a dressing, or manipulate equipment.

Implementation Methods

Assisting With ADLs

The nurse helps the patient perform activities and tasks that are performed in a normal day, such as bathing, dressing, and brushing teeth. The need for assistance with ADLs can be acute, chronic, temporary, permanent, or rehabilitative. For example, a postoperative patient may need assistance acutely for only 1 or 2 days after surgery. This is in contrast with a patient who has had a cerebrovascular accident and requires long-term, rehabilitative assistance. From the nursing assessment, the nurse can identify the amount of assistance needed for ADLs.

Counseling

The nurse helps the patient with problem solving and stress management by providing emotional, intellectual, spiritual, and psychological support. Counseling techniques used by the nurse promote a person's cognitive, behavioral, developmental, experiential, and emotional growth. They enable a patient to examine choices and thus gain a sense of control. To be effective, the nurse needs to develop a therapeutic relationship with the patient through the use of interpersonal skills.

Among the patients who need counseling are those who require lifestyle changes, such as smoking cessation, weight reduction, and decreasing activity levels. Also, patients who have chronic or disabling diseases need counseling to assist with the lifestyle changes and body image disturbances that they may encounter.

Patients and their families frequently need counseling when faced with death. The following counseling strategies are used by nurses:

- Behavior modification
- Bereavement counseling
- Biofeedback
- Relaxation training
- Reality orientation
- Crisis intervention
- Guided imagery
- Play therapy

Teaching

The nurse presents correct information about principles, procedures, and techniques to the patient. When providing education, the nurse must first assess the patient's learning needs, level of education, and motivation to learn.

Teaching and counseling are closely associated, in that they both involve communication skills to provide the patient with the tools needed to make a change. Teaching should be an ongoing process that builds on a person's knowledge base.

Performing Nursing Care Duties

The nurse needs to draw on his or her training and experience to perform specific care duties efficiently, smoothly, and accurately. These duties include the following:

- Evaluation and treatment of adverse reactions. An adverse reaction is a harmful or unintended effect of a medication or procedure. The nurse needs to know the potential undesired side effects to compensate for them, resulting in a reduction or an alleviation of the effects. For example, a nurse administering heparin should know that protamine sulfate will reverse the effects of heparin if bleeding problems result from its use.
- Preventive measures. Preventive nursing actions are aimed at preventing illness and promoting health.

Examples are assessment of the patient's health potential, health teaching, early diagnosis, and development of rehabilitation potential. The goal of preventive health measures is for the patient to achieve optimal wellness.
- Correct techniques in administering care and preparing a patient for procedures. The nurse needs knowledge and experience to carry out such procedures as changing dressings, inserting an indwelling catheter, and administering medications.
- Lifesaving measures. The purpose of a lifesaving measure is to restore physiologic or psychological stability, such as performing cardiopulmonary resuscitation, administering emergency medications, and restraining a violent patient. This type of intervention may be independent or collaborative.

Assisting the Patient to Attain Health Care Goals

The nurse adjusts care according to the patient's needs, stimulating and motivating the patient to achieve self-care and independence and encouraging the patient to accept care or follow the prescribed treatment regimen. In addition, the nurse and patient collaborate to achieve the goals they have developed together. Several methods can be used by the nurse to ensure that the patient achieves his or her goals.
- Provide the patient with enough privacy to meet basic needs but also be able to interact with the health care team. Orienting the patient to the health care facility fosters this independence and interaction.
- Provide for flexible, incremental, and attainable goals that the patient can successfully complete. With each level of independence a patient achieves, he or she goes on to the next level with more confidence in the ability to manage self-care requirements.
- Provide for adequate discharge planning and teaching to promote adherence to the treatment plan. The nurse needs to evaluate resources (personal and financial, for example) to promote a smooth transition to home.

For example, a cardiac patient with a two-story home may need a new home or some adjustments in his or her current home because of an inability to manage stairs. If this is not addressed before discharge, the patient may not adhere to the treatment plan. Counseling will help the patient and family make the changes needed because of the disease process or treatment.

Documentation

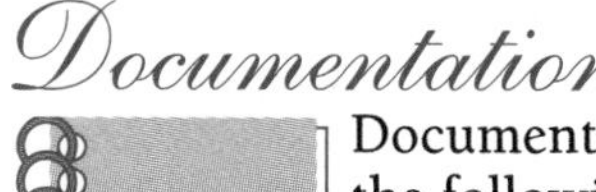

Documentation of nursing interventions is important for the following reasons:

- The patient's chart is a legal record of health care received.
- "If it is not recorded, it was not done."
- When a patient achieves his or her optimal level of wellness, the record shows the contribution that the nurse has made in this process.

It is important that the nurse document the following information objectively and concisely, using appropriate medical terminology:

- Date and time of the intervention
- Effectiveness of the intervention in achieving the proposed outcome
- Patient's progress toward resolution of the problem as stated in the nursing diagnosis

Suggested Readings

Ackerman, L. "Interventions Related to Neurologic Care." *Nursing Clinics of North America* 27, no.2 (1992): 325–347.

Brown, M. "How Do You Spell Assessment?...Simple Mnemonic Device to Organize Your Work." *American Journal of Nursing* 91 (September 1991): 55–56.

Bulechek, G. M., and J. C. McCloskey. "Defining and Validating Nursing Interventions." *Nursing Clinics of North America* 27, no. 2 (1992): 289–300.

Craft, M. J., and J. A. Willadsen. "Interventions Related to Family." *Nursing Clinics of North America* 27, no. 2 (1992): 517–540.

Hartman, D., and J. Knudson. "Documentation: A Nursing Data Base for Initial Patient Assessment." *Oncology Nursing Forum* 18 (January/February 1991): 125–130.

Hartrick, G., A. E. Lindsey, and M. Hills. "Family Nursing Assessment: Meeting the Challenge of Health Promotion." *Journal of Advanced Nursing* 20 (July 1994): 85–91.

Herr, K. A., and P. R. Mobily. “Interventions Related to Pain.” *Nursing Clinics of North America* 27, no. 2 (1992): 347–371.

Loos, F., and J. Bell. “Circular Questions: A Family Interviewing Strategy.” *Dimensions in Critical Care Nursing* 9, no. 1 (1990): 46–53.

Nelson, D. M. “Interventions Related to Respiratory Care.” *Nursing Clinics of North America* 27, no. 2 (1992): 301–324.

Rakel, B. A. “Interventions Related to Patient Teaching.” *Nursing Clinics of North America* 27, no. 2 (1992): 397–425.

Simons, M. R. “Interventions Related to Compliance.” *Nursing Clinics of North America* 27, no. 2 (1992): 477–495.

SECTION II. CHRONIC OBSTRUCTIVE PULMONARY DISEASES

Chapter 3. Bronchitis and Emphysema

▽ ▽ ▽ ▽ ▽ ▽ ▽

Introduction

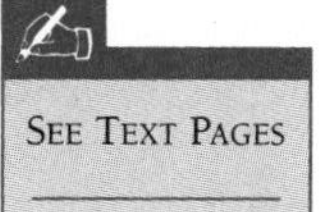

Bronchitis and emphysema are chronic obstructive pulmonary diseases. The term chronic obstructive pulmonary disease (COPD) is the general term used to denote a group of respiratory diseases whose primary characteristic is impaired lung function caused by small airway obstruction.

Chronic bronchitis is characterized by excessive production of mucus in the bronchi, causing chronic cough. To be considered chronic, these factors must be present for at least 3 months of the year for at least 2 years. The onset of symptoms may be insidious, and the patient may attribute many of them to the natural process of aging.

Emphysema is characterized by a loss of lung tissue elasticity and the abnormal enlargement of the alveolar ducts and alveoli to the point of destruction of the alveolar walls. Because the lungs' capacity to adequately exchange gases is impaired, patients who suffer from emphysema struggle to inhale more air. There are two primary types of emphysema: centrilobular and panlobular.

CHEST PERCUSSION AND POSTURAL DRAINAGE TECHNIQUES

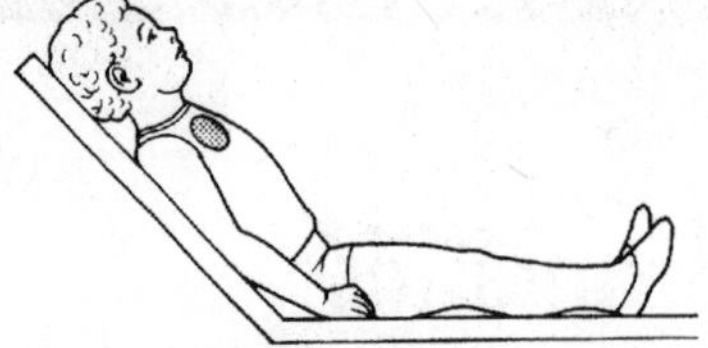

Apical segments–right and left upper lobes. *Torso elevated 30°.*

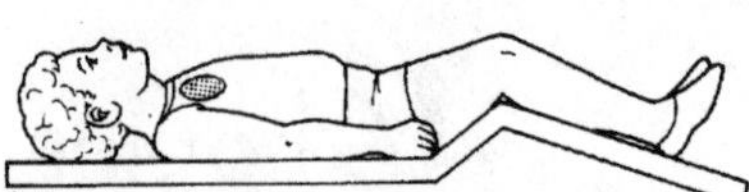

Anterior segments–right and left upper lobes. *Patient supine.*

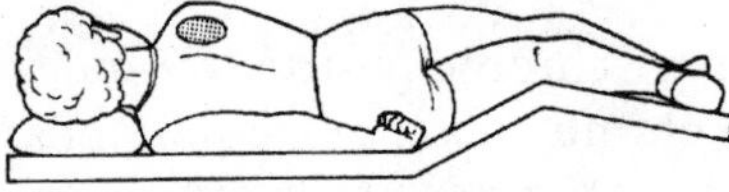

Posterior segment–right upper lobe. *Right side elevated 45°. Patient prone.*

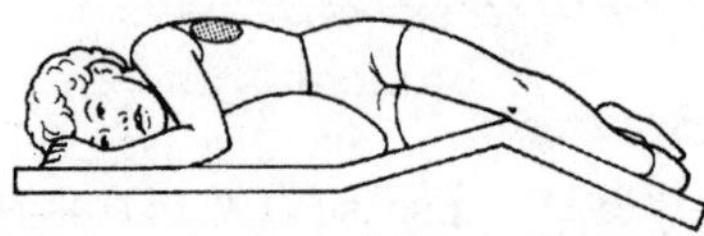

Posterior segment–left upper lobe. *Head elevated 15°. Left side elevated 45°.*

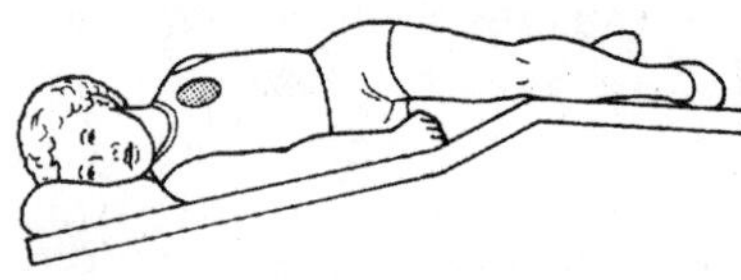

Lingular segment–left side. *Head lowered 15°. Patient on right hip, shoulders flat.*

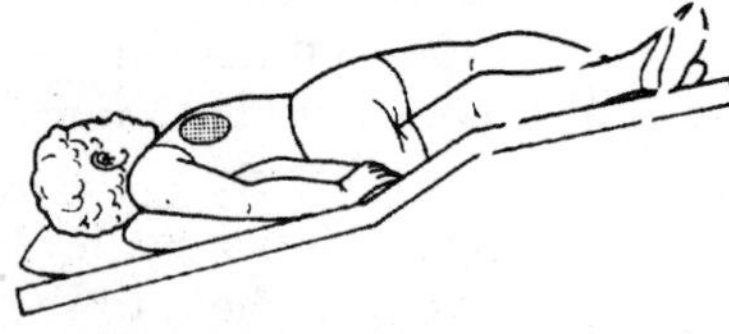

Right middle lobe. *Head lowered 15°. Right side elevated 45°.*

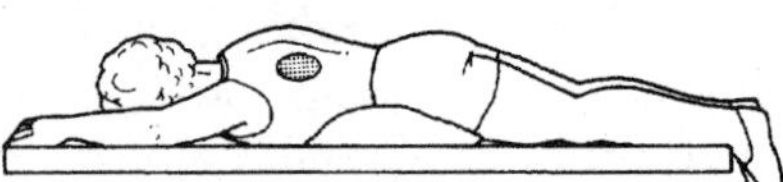

Apical segments–right and left lower lobes. *Patient prone.*

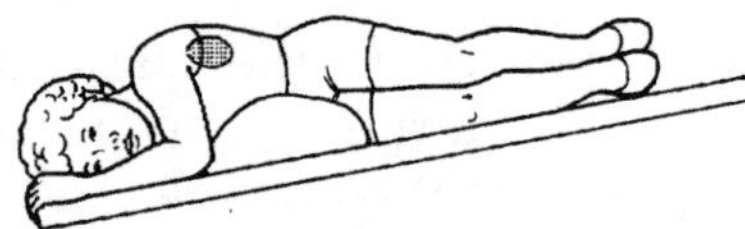

Lateral basal segment–left lower lobe. *Head lowered 30°. Left side elevated 45°.*

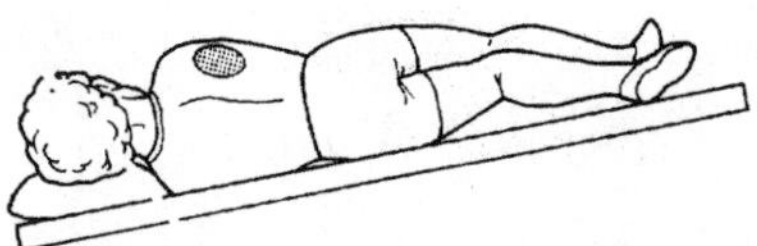

Lateral basal segment–right lower lobe. *Head lowered 30°. Right side elevated 45°.*

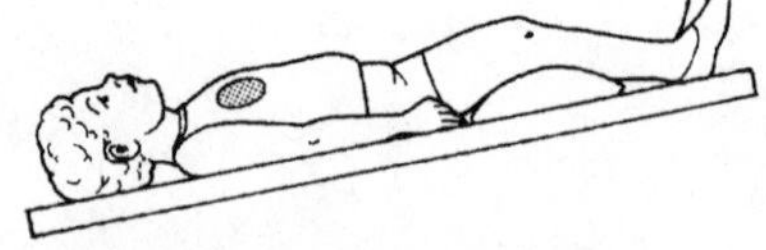

Anterior basal segments–right and left lower lobes. *Head lowered 30°. Patient supine.*

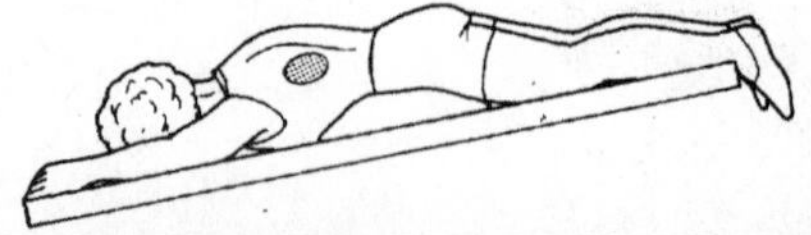

Posterior basal segments–right and left lower lobes. *Head lowered 30°. Patient prone.*

NURSING DIAGNOSES: IMPAIRED GAS EXCHANGE
INEFFECTIVE AIRWAY CLEARANCE
INEFFECTIVE BREATHING PATTERN

RELATED TO:

- *Increase in excessive mucus production, impaired ciliary movement, and chronic tissue hypoxia*

Nursing Interventions	Rationales
• Monitor respiratory status (for rate, effort, and breath sounds) and vital signs. Assess every 15 minutes to every several hours, depending on patient status.	• To identify impending respiratory failure
• Elevate the patient's head and back (high Fowler's position), and arrange pillows to support the patient's respiratory efforts.	• To facilitate diaphragmatic excursion, keep the airway open, and alleviate discomfort during breathing
• Encourage the patient to expectorate secretions or perform suction, if needed.	• To clear blockage from respiratory passageways
• Document the color, consistency, and amount of secretions.	• To determine the effectiveness of treatment
• Teach the patient breathing exercises, such as incentive spirometry.	• To open alveolar passages and increase sputum expectoration
• Assist in performing chest physiotherapy, as needed.	• To help mobilize and eliminate lung secretions
• Encourage the patient to drink adequate amounts of fluid, at least 1,500 to 2,000 mL daily, unless the patient's fluid intake has been restricted.	• To help loosen secretions and compensate for fluid loss from secretion expectoration and elevated temperature

NURSING DIAGNOSES: IMPAIRED GAS EXCHANGE *(CONTINUED)*

COLLABORATIVE MANAGEMENT

Interventions	Rationales
• Administer oxygen, as ordered.	• To prevent tissue hypoxia

NURSE ALERT:
Limit the fraction of inspired oxygen concentrations to those that achieve PaO_2 levels of 55 to 70 mm Hg. Higher PaO_2 levels may override the hypoxic drive needed to allow patients with COPD to breathe.

Interventions	Rationales
• Administer medications, as ordered: antibiotics, antipyretics, bronchodilators, expectorants, steroids.	• To resolve respiratory congestion, reduce fever, and reduce or prevent infection
• Consult with the respiratory therapist for information about chest physiotherapy.	• To ensure that the patient is receiving maximum benefit from therapy

OUTCOME:

- The patient will be able to breathe easily and effectively, sustain adequate ventilation, and maintain arterial blood gas values within normal ranges.

EVALUATION CRITERIA:

- Respirations are even and bilateral.
- Edema of affected tissues is decreased.
- Decreased pain or discomfort is reported.
- Uvula is located at midline.
- Pulse oximetry levels are adequate.

NURSING DIAGNOSIS: HIGH RISK FOR INFECTION

RELATED TO:

- *Altered respiratory function and impaired nutritional status*

Nursing Interventions	Rationales
• Monitor vital signs for changes that indicate infection, such as elevated temperature and rapid heart rate.	• To prevent onset or worsening of infection
• Encourage the patient to drink fluids, maintain adequate nutrition, and rest frequently.	• To prevent onset or worsening of infection
• Teach the patient basic infection control practices, such as hand washing and avoidance of other infected people.	• To minimize risk of contracting infection

COLLABORATIVE MANAGEMENT

Interventions	Rationales
• Administer medications as ordered: antibiotics, antipyretics, antitussives, steroids.	• To reduce or eliminate fever and infection

NURSE ALERT:
Be careful to assess the patient for adverse reactions to drugs and food.

Interventions	Rationales
• Consult with the dietitian to develop a dietary plan for the patient.	• To ensure adequate nutrition to support the body's struggle to combat infection

NURSING DIAGNOSIS: HIGH RISK FOR INFECTION *(CONTINUED)*

OUTCOME:

- The patient will be free of signs of infection.

EVALUATION CRITERIA:

- Vital signs are normal.
- White blood cell count is normal.
- Sputum is clear upon expectoration.

NURSING DIAGNOSIS: ALTERED NUTRITION (LESS THAN BODY REQUIREMENTS)

RELATED TO:

- *Anorexia and increased energy expenditure secondary to increased effort required for breathing*

Nursing Interventions	Rationales
• Assess the patient's current nutritional status: height, weight, and condition of skin, hair, and nails.	• To determine baseline
• Monitor the patient's weight daily or weekly.	• To track the effectiveness of interventions
• Encourage the patient to consume smaller, more frequent meals and high-calorie, high-protein snacks.	• To promote the consumption of adequate levels of nutrition and to prevent tiring from increased effort required for eating

COLLABORATIVE MANAGEMENT

Interventions	Rationales
• Administer supplemental vitamins and minerals, as ordered.	• To ensure adequate nutrition
• Consult with the dietitian to develop a dietary plan for the patient.	• To ensure adequate nutrition

COLLABORATIVE MANAGEMENT *(CONTINUED)*

Interventions *(Continued)*	Rationales *(Continued)*
• Assist with alternative feeding methods, such as tube feedings and intravenous feedings.	• To ensure adequate nutrition

NURSE ALERT:
If the patient is being fed by an alternative method, ensure the patency of the access route, administer the prescribed formulas, and document the amounts, patient response, and laboratory values, as appropriate.

OUTCOME:	EVALUATION CRITERIA:
• The patient will receive adequate nutrition to support body requirements.	• Caloric intake is increased. • Body weight is maintained at or just above recommended levels. • Improvement in appetite is noted.

NURSING DIAGNOSIS: HIGH RISK FOR ACTIVITY INTOLERANCE

RELATED TO:
- *Dyspnea and fatigue*

Nursing Interventions	Rationales
• Plan patient care activities to take advantage of the patient's periods of energy.	• To avoid overtiring the patient

NURSING DIAGNOSIS: HIGH RISK FOR ACTIVITY INTOLERANCE (CONTINUED)

Nursing Interventions *(Continued)*	Rationales *(Continued)*
• Assist the patient in identifying his or her level of ability and point of fatigue.	• To encourage the patient to identify the need to get adequate rest
• Keep the patient's supplies, food, and possessions close at hand.	• To avoid increasing the patient's workload and to prevent additional exertion

COLLABORATIVE MANAGEMENT

Interventions	Rationales
• Consult with the physician and exercise physiologist to develop an exercise program for the patient..	• To increase the patient's stamina and work capacity

OUTCOME:	EVALUATION CRITERIA:
• The patient will be free from extended periods of extreme fatigue and will be able to perform activities of daily living with little effort or respiratory difficulty.	• Increased levels of activity are observed and reported. • The patient is able to complete activities of daily living.

NURSING DIAGNOSES: ANXIETY POWERLESSNESS

RELATED TO:

- *Uncertain outcome of the disorder, respiratory difficulties, and lack of information about the disorder, treatment plans, diagnostic tests, and procedures*

Nursing Interventions	Rationales
• Explain the condition to the patient and family members or other caregivers, using appropriate language for the patient's level of understanding.	• To ease unfamiliarity and discomfort and allow the patient some control over the situation

Nursing Interventions *(Continued)*	Rationales *(Continued)*
• Monitor the patient for signs of increasing distress, such as verbal or nonverbal communication.	• To prevent levels of anxiety and fear from becoming an additional burden on the patient's condition
• Maintain a calm, relaxed demeanor, and reassure the patient that his or her condition is being monitored at all times.	• To avoid additional anxiety concerning the staff's presence and attitude
• Encourage the patient to share his or her concerns, and respond to each as appropriate.	• To maintain open lines of communication
• Promote a quiet environment by reducing external stimulation.	• To limit the drain on the patient's resources—mental, emotional, and physical
• Plan care activities for times when the patient is feeling best able to handle the stress.	• To avoid unduly stressing the patient
• Encourage the patient to stop smoking and to ask other smokers to avoid smoking around him or her.	• To give the patient a means to exert some control over his or her condition
• Teach the patient about the role stress and emotions play in exacerbating infections and decreasing the body's ability to cope with illness.	• To promote the patient's control over his or her emotional well-being

COLLABORATIVE MANAGEMENT

Interventions	Rationales
• Administer medications, as ordered: sedatives.	• To decrease the patient's anxiety and fear

NURSING DIAGNOSES: ANXIETY *(CONTINUED)*

COLLABORATIVE MANAGEMENT *(CONTINUED)*

Interventions *(Continued)*	Rationales *(Continued)*
• Encourage the patient and family members to take advantage of counseling services and support groups, as appropriate.	• To develop effective coping skills

OUTCOME:	EVALUATION CRITERIA:
• The patient will appear calm and relaxed.	• Physical signs of distress, such as agitation, restlessness, and elevated respiratory rate are absent or decreased. • The patient reports that he or she is feeling more confident and relaxed.

NURSING DIAGNOSIS: KNOWLEDGE DEFICIT

RELATED TO:

- *Methods for delaying the progress of COPD, palliative measures, and maintaining optimum levels of health*

Nursing Interventions	Rationales
• Educate the patient about the pathophysiology of the disorder, prescribed medications and possible adverse effects, follow-up care requirements, and danger signs that should be reported to the health care provider.	• To increase the patient's understanding
• Include the patient's family and other caregivers in the educational program.	• To increase the likelihood that the patient will follow the self-care regimen

COLLABORATIVE MANAGEMENT

Interventions	Rationales
• Refer the patient, family, and other caregivers to the appropriate support agencies.	• To encourage understanding of the patient's condition
• Collaborate with other health care providers in stressing the importance of the health care regimen.	• To ensure understanding of the importance of the health care regimen

OUTCOME:

- The patient will demonstrate adequate knowledge about the disorder and self-care routines.

EVALUATION CRITERIA:

- The patient accurately describes the physical effects of the disorder.
- The patient verbalizes an understanding of the use of medications, their adverse effects, and danger signs.
- The patient complies with follow-up appointments and self-care regimen.
- The patient seeks health care, if conditions indicate the need.

NURSING DIAGNOSIS: NONCOMPLIANCE

RELATED TO:

- *Denial of the condition, difficulties involved in lifestyle changes required to accommodate the condition, and lack of knowledge about the disease and required changes*

Nursing Interventions	Rationales
• Determine the nature of the patient's noncompliance through discussion with the patient and his or her family or other caregivers, if possible and appropriate.	• To determine areas on which to focus your interventions

NURSING DIAGNOSIS: NONCOMPLIANCE *(CONTINUED)*

Nursing Interventions *(Continued)*	Rationales *(Continued)*
• Listen to the patient's reasons for noncompliance. Respond in a nonjudgmental manner.	• To encourage the patient to express his or her concerns and to emphasize that you respect the patient's opinions and right to make decisions about care and treatment
• Provide appropriate information about lifestyle changes, treatment options, the patient's condition, and coping techniques.	• To increase patient knowledge, which alleviates noncompliance due to lack of knowledge
• Develop a contract with the patient to identify tasks the patient will do, changes he or she will make (such as smoking cessation and weight management), and goals the patient will attempt to meet.	• To increase patient participation in acceptable activities, thereby increasing overall compliance

NURSE ALERT:
Remember that it is the patient's right to refuse treatment or to participate in a care plan and you must respect that right, provided it does not endanger you, other staff members, or other patients.

COLLABORATIVE MANAGEMENT

Interventions	Rationales
• Explain the patient's decisions to other staff members. Document the patient's decisions carefully.	• To identify the ways in which other staff members may have to alter their care plans and activities
• Collaborate with other health care providers in stressing the importance of the health care regimen.	• To ensure understanding of the importance of the health care regimen

COLLABORATIVE MANAGEMENT *(CONTINUED)*

Interventions *(Continued)*	Rationales *(Continued)*
• Encourage the patient to participate in discussions with other patients who are coping with the same problems, limitations, and challenges.	• To provide an opportunity for the patient to learn new methods for coping with bronchitis or emphysema and thereby increase the potential for patient compliance

OUTCOME:	EVALUATION CRITERIA:
• The patient will complete self-care activities and participate in treatment, as established by mutual agreement.	• The patient enters into a care and treatment contract. • The patient complies with follow-up appointments and self-care regimen, as defined.

NURSING DIAGNOSIS: SOCIAL ISOLATION

RELATED TO:

- *Embarrassment about dyspnea, coughing, related sputum expectoration, equipment required for treatment such as oxygen concentrators, restrictions on activity, and the withdrawal of friends and family members who are uncomfortable with the patient's disease*

Nursing Interventions	Rationales
• Discuss the changes in the patient's social activities that have been brought about the disease. Identify any misconceptions the patient might have.	• To promote expression of the patient's concerns and questions
• Explain that while the disease does impose limitation on the patient's physical activity, reasonable exertion and exercise may actually improve the patient's condition. Caution the patient about starting a cycle of exercise avoidance, which leads to intolerance.	• To encourage the patient to remain as physically active as possible

NURSING DIAGNOSIS: SOCIAL ISOLATION *(CONTINUED)*

Nursing Interventions *(Continued)*	Rationales *(Continued)*
• Educate the patient and his or her family and caregivers about the condition, its treatment requirements, and ways in which the patient can remain an active participant in many social activities.	• To increase patient and family understanding
• Encourage the patient to maintain and develop a network of friends and acquaintances with whom he or she can communicate frequently, in person, over the phone, by letter, or using the computer.	• To develop additional outlets for social expression for the patient

COLLABORATIVE MANAGEMENT

Interventions	Rationales
• Encourage the patient to discuss, with appropriate therapists, the choices for any medical equipment. Emphasize that many units are portable and unobtrusive.	• To provide options for the patient to consider
• Identify support groups and other resources the patient can contact for information and advice, such as the American Lung Association.	• To promote the development of a support network
• Refer the patient to appropriate counseling to discuss issues related to social isolation and loneliness.	• To provide an additional outlet for the patient to express his or her feelings, fears, and concerns

NURSING DIAGNOSIS: SOCIAL ISOLATION *(CONTINUED)*

OUTCOME:

- The patient will participate in social activities, as appropriate for his or her condition.

EVALUATION CRITERIA:

- The patient expresses satisfaction with the social activities in which he or she is engaged.
- The patient takes appropriate measures to promote his or her participation in social activities, such as engaging in an exercise program to build stamina.

Patient Teaching

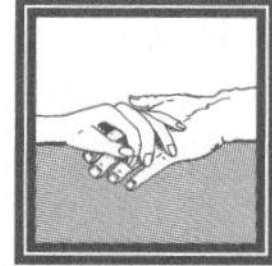

Patient teaching should center around ways to cope with the physical and psychosocial limitations imposed by chronic bronchitis, ease the symptoms of the disorder, and prevent further disability, as well as the importance of self-care regimens.

Instruct the patient about the role smoking plays in COPD. Encourage the patient to stop smoking by providing educational information and referrals to smoking cessation programs.

Teach the patient about tips and techniques for making everyday tasks easier. For example, suggest that the patient rest before preparing and eating meals to avoid bouts of dyspnea and that he or she move commonly used items to easy-to-reach areas to avoid overexertion. Advise the patient to schedule errands and other tasks for asymptomatic periods to help reduce physical and emotional stress.

Encourage the patient and his or her family to express their thoughts and concerns about the disorder. Refer them to appropriate counseling agencies, if needed. Reinforce the importance of using previously effective coping skills, developing new skills, and setting realistic goals to deal with the anxiety, stress, and depression that may accompany the disorder. Involve family members and other potential caregivers in the educational program as much as possible. Stress the importance of promoting wellness, as opposed to concentrating on the patient's sickness.

Teach the patient about proper bronchial hygiene, including hydration, humidification of inspired air, and postural drainage.

Instruct the patient to perform pursed-lip breathing and diaphragmatic breathing. Both help to slow the respiratory rate and promote effective coughing.

Pursed-lip breathing requires the patient to inhale slowly through the nose and exhale more slowly through the mouth. The lips should be positioned as if the patient were whistling. Exhalation should last twice as long as inhalation. This helps to prevent air from becoming trapped in the collapsed bronchioles.

Diaphragmatic breathing requires the patient to use the diaphragm to slow the respiratory rate and increase the depth of inhalation. Instruct the patient to place one hand on the abdomen and the other hand on the apical area of the chest. The patient then inhales slowly through the nose. When the diaphragm is used properly to control respiration, the hand resting on the abdomen should rise and the hand resting on the chest should remain still.

Inform the patient about immunization against pneumococcal infection and influenza. Because infections can cause exacerbation of symptoms, it is important that the patient take steps to reduce the risk of infection and to treat colds and flu quickly.

Instruct the patient about the proper use of bronchodilators and the use of various medications to control the symptoms of the disorder.

Discuss the importance of maintaining weight at or just under the target weight.

Teach the patient and family members about the disorder and the importance of the therapeutic regimen, especially exercise programs designed to improve endurance and increase the efficiency of the respiratory muscles, breathing retraining, adequate nutrition, and psychosocial support.

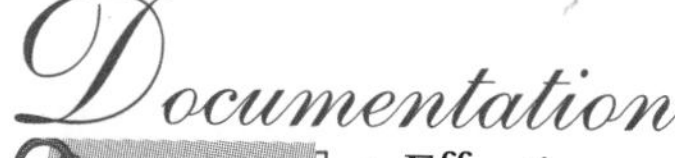

Documentation

- Effectiveness of therapeutic measures
- Vital signs, weight, and skin, nail, and hair condition
- Patient intake and output, especially caloric intake

Nursing Research

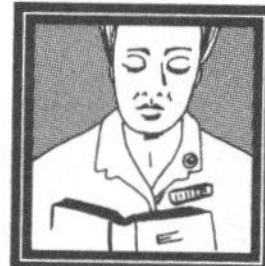

Studies show that patient education is a key element in successful management of chronic bronchitis. In a 1987 study, Howard, Davies, and Roghmann found that participation in a structured teaching program reduced the number of hospital stays and increased the length of time between stays. Patient education should be patient-focused and appropriate to the patient's level of understanding and should include reinforcement and return of information by the patient.

Brundage, Dorothy J., Phyllis Swearengen, and Johnsie W. Woody. "Self-Care Instruction for Patients with COPD." *Rehabilitation Nursing* 18 (September/October 1993): 321–324.

Chapter 4. Bronchiectasis

▽ ▽ ▽ ▽ ▽ ▽ ▽

Introduction

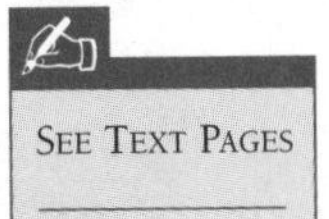

Bronchiectasis is a condition in which the bronchial walls, weakened by damage to the mucosa and the muscle walls, become permanently dilated. Purulent secretions collect in the dilated areas. Chronic infection results, further weakening the bronchioles and perpetuating the condition.

Bronchiectasis may be caused by aspiration of purulent mucus, inhalation of a foreign body, complications of cystic fibrosis, or other pulmonary infections.

NURSING DIAGNOSES: IMPAIRED GAS EXCHANGE
INEFFECTIVE AIRWAY CLEARANCE
INEFFECTIVE BREATHING PATTERN

RELATED TO:

- *Increase in excessive mucus production, impaired ciliary movement, and chronic tissue hypoxia*

Nursing Interventions	Rationales
• Monitor respiratory status (for rate, effort, and breath sounds) and vital signs. Assess every 15 minutes to every several hours, depending on patient status.	• To identify impending respiratory failure
• Elevate the patient's head and back (high Fowler's position), and arrange pillows to support the patient's respiratory efforts.	• To facilitate diaphragmatic excursion, keep the airway open, and alleviate discomfort during breathing
• Encourage the patient to expectorate secretions or perform suction, if needed.	• To clear blockage from respiratory passageways
• Document the color, consistency, and amount of secretions.	• To determine the effectiveness of treatment

Nursing Interventions *(Continued)*	Rationales *(Continued)*
• Teach the patient breathing exercises, such as incentive spirometry.	• To open alveolar passages and increase sputum expectoration
• Assist in performing chest physiotherapy, as needed.	• To help mobilize and eliminate lung secretions
• Encourage the patient to drink adequate amounts of fluid, at least 1,500 to 2,000 mL daily, unless the patient's fluid intake has been restricted.	• To help loosen secretions and compensate for fluid loss from secretion expectoration and elevated temperature

COLLABORATIVE MANAGEMENT

Interventions	Rationales
• Administer oxygen, as ordered.	• To prevent tissue hypoxia

NURSE ALERT:
Limit the fraction of inspired oxygen concentrations to those that achieve PaO_2 levels of 55 to 70 mm Hg. Higher PaO_2 levels may override the hypoxic drive needed to allow patients with COPD to breathe.

Interventions	Rationales
• Administer medications, as ordered: antibiotics, antipyretics, bronchodilators, expectorants, steroids.	• To resolve respiratory congestion, reduce fever, and reduce or prevent infection
• Consult with the respiratory therapist for information about chest physiotherapy.	• To ensure that the patient is receiving maximum benefit from therapy

NURSING DIAGNOSES: IMPAIRED GAS EXCHANGE *(CONTINUED)*

OUTCOME:

- The patient will be able to breathe easily and effectively, sustain adequate ventilation, and maintain arterial blood gas values within normal ranges.

EVALUATION CRITERIA:

- Respirations are even and bilateral.
- Edema of affected tissues is decreased.
- Decreased pain or discomfort is reported.
- Uvula is located at midline.
- Pulse oximetry levels are adequate.

NURSING DIAGNOSIS: HIGH RISK FOR INFECTION

RELATED TO:

- *Altered respiratory function and impaired nutritional status*

Nursing Interventions	Rationales
• Monitor vital signs for changes that indicate infection, such as elevated temperature and rapid heart rate.	• To prevent onset or worsening of infection
• Encourage the patient to drink fluids, maintain adequate nutrition, and rest frequently.	• To prevent onset or worsening of infection
• Teach the patient basic infection control practices, such as hand washing and avoidance of other infected people.	• To minimize risk of contracting infection

COLLABORATIVE MANAGEMENT

Interventions	Rationales
• Administer medications as ordered: antibiotics, antipyretics, antitussives, steroids.	• To reduce or eliminate fever and infection

NURSE ALERT:
Be careful to assess the patient for adverse reactions to drugs and food.

Interventions	Rationales
• Consult with the dietitian to develop a dietary plan for the patient.	• To ensure adequate nutrition to support the body's struggle to combat infection

OUTCOME:

- The patient will be free of signs of infection.

EVALUATION CRITERIA:

- Vital signs are normal.
- White blood cell count is normal.
- Sputum is clear upon expectoration.

NURSING DIAGNOSES: ANXIETY POWERLESSNESS

RELATED TO:

- *Uncertain outcome of the disorder, respiratory difficulties, and lack of information about the disorder, treatment plans, diagnostic tests, and procedures*

Nursing Interventions	Rationales
• Explain the condition to the patient and family members or other caregivers, using appropriate language for the patient's level of understanding.	• To ease unfamiliarity and discomfort and allow the patient some control over the situation

NURSING DIAGNOSES: ANXIETY *(CONTINUED)*

Nursing Interventions *(Continued)*	Rationales *(Continued)*
• Monitor the patient for signs of increasing distress, such as verbal or nonverbal communication.	• To prevent levels of anxiety and fear from becoming an additional burden on the patient's condition
• Maintain a calm, relaxed demeanor, and reassure the patient that his or her condition is being monitored at all times.	• To avoid additional anxiety concerning the staff's presence and attitude
• Encourage the patient to share his or her concerns, and respond to each as appropriate.	• To maintain open lines of communication
• Promote a quiet environment by reducing external stimulation.	• To limit the drain on the patient's resources—mental, emotional, and physical
• Plan care activities for times when the patient is feeling best able to handle the stress.	• To avoid unduly stressing the patient
• Encourage the patient to stop smoking and to ask other smokers to avoid smoking around him or her.	• To give the patient a means to exert some control over his or her condition
• Teach the patient about the role stress and emotions play in exacerbating infections and decreasing the body's ability to cope with illness.	• To promote the patient's control over his or her emotional well-being

COLLABORATIVE MANAGEMENT

Interventions	Rationales
• Administer medications, as ordered: sedatives.	• To decrease the patient's anxiety and fear
• Encourage the patient and family members to take advantage of counseling services and support groups, as appropriate.	• To develop effective coping skills

NURSING DIAGNOSES: ANXIETY *(CONTINUED)*

OUTCOME:	EVALUATION CRITERIA:
• The patient will appear calm and relaxed.	• Physical signs of distress, such as agitation, restlessness, and elevated respiratory rate are absent or decreased.
	• The patient reports that he or she is feeling more confident and relaxed.

NURSING DIAGNOSIS: KNOWLEDGE DEFICIT

RELATED TO:

- *Methods for disease state, palliative measures, and maintaining optimum levels of health*

Nursing Interventions	Rationales
• Educate the patient about the pathophysiology of the disorder, prescribed medications and possible adverse effects, follow-up care requirements, and danger signs that should be reported to the health care provider.	• To increase the patient's understanding • To increase the likelihood that the patient will follow the self-care regimen
• Include the patient's family and other caregivers in the educational program.	

COLLABORATIVE MANAGEMENT

Interventions	Rationales
• Refer the patient, family, and other caregivers to the appropriate support agencies.	• To encourage understanding of the patient's condition
• Collaborate with other health care providers in stressing the importance of the health care regimen.	• To ensure understanding of the importance of the health care regimen

NURSING DIAGNOSIS: KNOWLEDGE DEFICIT *(CONTINUED)*

OUTCOME:

- The patient will demonstrate adequate knowledge about the disorder and self-care routines.

EVALUATION CRITERIA:

- The patient accurately describes the physical effects of the disorder.
- The patient verbalizes an understanding of the use of medications, their adverse effects, and danger signs.
- The patient complies with follow-up appointments and self-care regimen.
- The patient seeks health care, if conditions indicate the need.

Patient Teaching

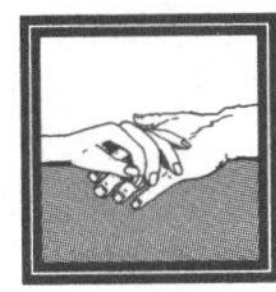

Emphasize the importance of treating any infections quickly and thoroughly. The patient should take steps to reduce the risk of infection, such as avoiding people with other infections such as colds of influenza, adhering to strict infection control measures, and seeking immunization against pneumococcal infection and influenza.

Teach the patient about proper bronchial hygiene, including hydration and humidification of inspired air. Explain changes the patient can make in his or her environment to reduce exacerbation of the illness, such as eliminating fumes or other irritants caused by products such as oven cleaners, air fresheners, or insect sprays.

Explain postural drainage procedures that the patient should use on a regular basis, to promote elimination of secretions. Percussion may help to loosen secretions and facilitate removal. Instruct the patient and his or her caregiver to exercise caution when performing percussion, especially if the patient is physically frail or at risk for brittle bones.

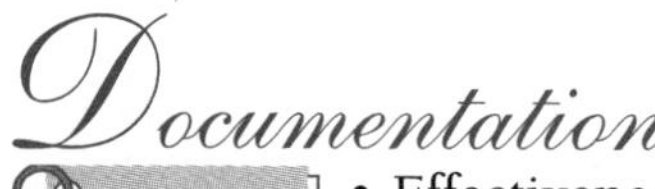

Documentation

- Effectiveness of therapeutic measures
- Patient vital signs, weight, and skin, nail, and hair condition
- Patient intake and output, especially caloric intake

Chapter 5. Cystic Fibrosis

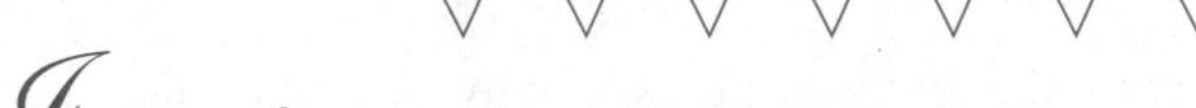

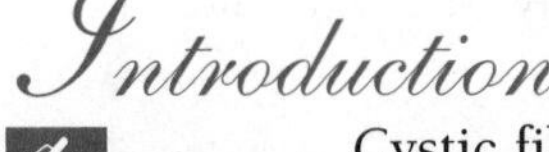

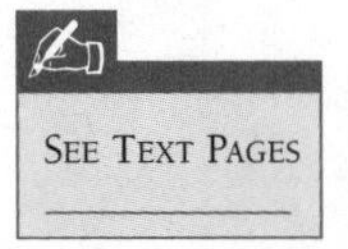

Cystic fibrosis is a hereditary disease in which mucus normally produced by the exocrine glands is abnormally viscid. It occurs in about 1 in 2,000 births. The disease is usually discovered and diagnosed in children and patients rarely live beyond their early 20's.

NURSING DIAGNOSES: IMPAIRED GAS EXCHANGE
INEFFECTIVE AIRWAY CLEARANCE
INEFFECTIVE BREATHING PATTERN

RELATED TO:

- *Increase in excessive mucus production, impaired ciliary movement, and chronic tissue hypoxia*

Nursing Interventions	Rationales
• Monitor respiratory status (for rate, effort, and breath sounds) and vital signs. Assess every 15 minutes to every several hours, depending on patient status.	• To identify impending respiratory failure
• Elevate the patient's head and back (high Fowler's position), and arrange pillows to support the patient's respiratory efforts.	• To facilitate diaphragmatic excursion, keep the airway open, and alleviate discomfort during breathing
• Encourage the patient to expectorate secretions or perform suction, if needed.	• To clear blockage from respiratory passageways
• Document the color, consistency, and amount of secretions.	• To determine the effectiveness of treatment
• Teach the patient breathing exercises, such as incentive spirometry.	• To open alveolar passages and increase sputum expectoration

Nursing Interventions *(Continued)*	Rationales *(Continued)*
• Assist in performing chest physiotherapy, as needed.	• To help mobilize and eliminate lung secretions
• Encourage the patient to drink adequate amounts of fluid, at least 1,500 to 2,000 mL daily, unless the patient's fluid intake has been restricted.	• To help loosen secretions and compensate for fluid loss from secretion expectoration and elevated temperature

COLLABORATIVE MANAGEMENT

Interventions	Rationales
• Administer oxygen, as ordered.	• To prevent tissue hypoxia

NURSE ALERT:
Limit the fraction of inspired oxygen concentrations to those that achieve Pao_2 levels of 55 to 70 mm Hg. Higher Pao_2 levels may override the hypoxic drive needed to allow patients with COPD to breathe.

Interventions	Rationales
• Administer medications, as ordered: antibiotics, antipyretics, bronchodilators, expectorants, steroids.	• To resolve respiratory congestion, reduce fever, and reduce or prevent infection
• Consult with the respiratory therapist for information about chest physiotherapy.	• To ensure that the patient is receiving maximum benefit from therapy

NURSING DIAGNOSES: IMPAIRED GAS EXCHANGE *(CONTINUED)*

OUTCOME:	EVALUATION CRITERIA:
• The patient will be able to breathe easily and effectively, sustain adequate ventilation, and maintain arterial blood gas values within normal ranges.	• Respirations are even and bilateral. • Edema of affected tissues is decreased. • Decreased pain or discomfort is reported. • Uvula is located at midline. • Pulse oximetry levels are adequate.

NURSING DIAGNOSIS: HIGH RISK FOR INFECTION

RELATED TO:

• *Altered respiratory function and impaired nutritional status*

Nursing Interventions	Rationales
• Monitor vital signs for changes that indicate infection, such as elevated temperature and rapid heart rate.	• To prevent onset or worsening of infection
• Encourage the patient to drink fluids, maintain adequate nutrition, and rest frequently.	• To prevent onset or worsening of infection
• Teach the patient basic infection control practices, such as hand washing and avoidance of other infected people.	• To minimize risk of contracting infection

COLLABORATIVE MANAGEMENT

Interventions	Rationales
• Administer medications as ordered: antibiotics, antipyretics, antitussives, steroids.	• To reduce or eliminate fever and infection

NURSE ALERT:
Be careful to assess the patient for adverse reactions to drugs and food.

• Consult with the dietitian to develop a dietary plan for the patient.	• To ensure adequate nutrition to support the body's struggle to combat infection

OUTCOME:	EVALUATION CRITERIA:
• The patient will be free of signs of infection.	• Vital signs are normal. • White blood cell count is normal. • Sputum is clear upon expectoration.

NURSING DIAGNOSIS: ALTERED NUTRITION (LESS THAN BODY REQUIREMENTS)

RELATED TO:

- *Anorexia and increased energy expenditure secondary to increased effort required for breathing*

Nursing Interventions	Rationales
• Assess the patient's current nutritional status: height, weight, and condition of skin, hair, and nails.	• To determine baseline
• Monitor the patient's weight daily or weekly.	• To track the effectiveness of interventions

NURSING DIAGNOSIS: ALTERED NUTRITION (LESS THAN BODY REQUIREMENTS) *(CONTINUED)*

Nursing Interventions *(Continued)*	Rationales *(Continued)*
• Encourage the patient to consume smaller, more frequent meals and high-calorie, high-protein snacks.	• To promote the consumption of adequate levels of nutrition and to prevent tiring from increased effort required for eating

COLLABORATIVE MANAGEMENT

Interventions	Rationales
• Administer supplemental vitamins and minerals, as ordered.	• To ensure adequate nutrition
• Consult with the dietitian to develop a dietary plan for the patient.	• To ensure adequate nutrition
• Assist with alternative feeding methods, such as tube feedings and intravenous feedings.	• To ensure adequate nutrition

NURSE ALERT:
If the patient is being fed by an alternative method, ensure the patency of the access route, administer the prescribed formulas, and document the amounts, patient response, and laboratory values, as appropriate.

OUTCOME:	EVALUATION CRITERIA:
• The patient will receive adequate nutrition to support body requirements.	• Caloric intake is increased.
	• Body weight is maintained at or just above recommended levels.
	• Improvement in appetite is noted.

NURSING DIAGNOSIS: HIGH RISK FOR ACTIVITY INTOLERANCE

RELATED TO:

- *Dyspnea and fatigue*

Nursing Interventions	Rationales
• Plan patient care activities to take advantage of the patient's periods of energy.	• To avoid overtiring the patient

NURSE ALERT:
Generally, early morning and just after mealtime are not good times for patient care activities. In the morning, the patient will need to expend additional energy to clear nighttime secretions. After a meal, the patient will usually experience abdominal distention, putting a limit on diaphragmatic excursion, which increases breathing effort.

Nursing Interventions	Rationales
• Assist the patient in identifying his or her level of ability and point of fatigue.	• To encourage the patient to identify the need to get adequate rest
• Keep the patient's supplies, food, and possessions close at hand.	• To avoid increasing the patient's workload and to prevent additional exertion

COLLABORATIVE MANAGEMENT

Interventions	Rationales
• Consult with the physician and exercise physiologist to develop an exercise program for the patient.	• To increase the patient's stamina and work capacity

NURSING DIAGNOSIS: HIGH RISK FOR ACTIVITY INTOLERANCE *(CONTINUED)*

OUTCOME:

- The patient will be free from extended periods of extreme fatigue and will be able to perform activities of daily living with little effort or respiratory difficulty.

EVALUATION CRITERIA:

- Increased levels of activity are observed and reported.
- The patient is able to complete activities of daily living.

NURSING DIAGNOSES: ANXIETY POWERLESSNESS

RELATED TO:

- *Uncertain outcome of the disorder, respiratory difficulties, and lack of information about the disorder, treatment plans, diagnostic tests, and procedures*

Nursing Interventions	Rationales
• Explain the condition to the patient and family members or other caregivers, using appropriate language for the patient's level of understanding.	• To ease unfamiliarity and discomfort and allow the patient some control over the situation
• Monitor the patient for signs of increasing distress, such as verbal or nonverbal communication.	• To prevent levels of anxiety and fear from becoming an additional burden on the patient's condition
• Maintain a calm, relaxed demeanor, and reassure the patient that his or her condition is being monitored at all times.	• To avoid additional anxiety concerning the staff's presence and attitude
• Encourage the patient to share his or her concerns, and respond to each as appropriate.	• To maintain open lines of communication
• Promote a quiet environment by reducing external stimulation.	• To limit the drain on the patient's resources—mental, emotional, and physical

Nursing Interventions *(Continued)*	Rationales *(Continued)*
• Plan care activities for times when the patient is feeling best able to handle the stress.	• To avoid unduly stressing the patient
• Encourage the patient to stop smoking and to ask other smokers to avoid smoking around him or her.	• To give the patient a means to exert some control over his or her condition
• Teach the patient about the role stress and emotions play in exacerbating infections and decreasing the body's ability to cope with illness.	• To promote the patient's control over his or her emotional well-being

COLLABORATIVE MANAGEMENT

Interventions	Rationales
• Administer medications, as ordered: sedatives.	• To decrease the patient's anxiety and fear
• Encourage the patient and family members to take advantage of counseling services and support groups, as appropriate.	• To develop effective coping skills

OUTCOME:	EVALUATION CRITERIA:
• The patient will appear calm and relaxed.	• Physical signs of distress, such as agitation, restlessness, and elevated respiratory rate are absent or decreased. • The patient reports that he or she is feeling more confident and relaxed.

NURSING DIAGNOSIS: KNOWLEDGE DEFICIT

RELATED TO:

- *Methods for delaying the progress of COPD, palliative measures, and maintaining optimum levels of health*

Nursing Interventions	Rationales
• Educate the patient about the pathophysiology of the disorder, prescribed medications and possible adverse effects, follow-up care requirements, and danger signs that should be reported to the health care provider.	• To increase the patient's understanding
• Include the patient's family and other caregivers in the educational program.	• To increase the likelihood that the patient will follow the self-care regimen

COLLABORATIVE MANAGEMENT

Interventions	Rationales
• Refer the patient, family, and other caregivers to the appropriate support agencies.	• To encourage understanding of the patient's condition
• Collaborate with other health care providers in stressing the importance of the health care regimen.	• To ensure understanding of the importance of the health care regimen

OUTCOME:

- The patient will demonstrate adequate knowledge about the disorder and self-care routines.

EVALUATION CRITERIA:

- The patient accurately describes the physical effects of the disorder.
- The patient verbalizes an understanding of the use of medications, their adverse effects, and danger signs.
- The patient complies with follow-up appointments and self-care regimen.
- The patient seeks health care, if conditions indicate the need.

NURSING DIAGNOSIS: INEFFECTIVE FAMILY COPING

RELATED TO:

- *Diagnosis of cystic fibrosis, prognosis, and death of family member*

Nursing Interventions	Rationales
• Explain the patient's condition to the family, and if appropriate, to the patient. Allow the family time to absorb the information. Answer questions and provide information as the family requests.	• To increase patient and family understanding

NURSE ALERT:
Often the family will request information you have already provided or ask the same questions repeatedly. Provide answers each time, taking into account that the information may not be completely absorbed or understood, as the family comes to terms with the situation.

Nursing Interventions	Rationales
• Emphasize that although the disease is a serious one, and that certain adaptations will have to be made to accommodate the patient's condition, the family should make every effort to lead a normal, active life.	• To help the family and patient maintain a realistic perspective and develop effective coping skills
• Encourage the family to discuss options for treatment, diagnostic procedures, and lifestyle changes with the patient.	• To encourage patient involvement in the care plan and to promote the development of effective coping skills by the whole family

NURSING DIAGNOSIS: INEFFECTIVE FAMILY COPING
(CONTINUED)

COLLABORATIVE MANAGEMENT

Interventions	Rationales
• Refer the patient, family, and other caregivers to the appropriate support agencies.	• To encourage understanding of the patient's condition
• Refer the family to appropriate financial consultants.	• To provide information about the financial arrangements that may be necessary, considering the long-term nature of the disease
• Encourage the family to pursue activities for other children in the family.	• To discourage unhealthy preoccupation with the illness and the sick family member

OUTCOME:	EVALUATION CRITERIA:
• The patient and family will come to terms with the diagnosis, the disease, and the required changes that will occur over time.	• The patient and family discuss care plans, diagnostic procedures, and the care regimen as appropriate. • Signs of disharmony, such as avoidance of the family member, excessive arguing, and ignoring of other family members, are absent. • The patient and family understand and comply with treatment requirements.

Patient Teaching

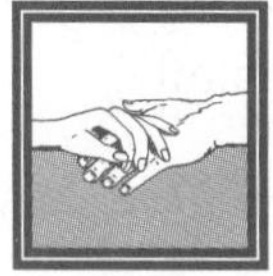

Patient teaching should center around ways to cope with the physical and psychosocial limitations imposed by cystic fibrosis. Emphasis should be placed on helping the family deal with the diagnosis, the severity of the illness, and the potential loss of a child.

Encourage the patient and his or her family to express their thoughts and concerns about the disorder. Refer them to appropriate counseling agencies, if needed. Reinforce the importance of using previously effective coping skills, developing new skills, and setting realistic goals to deal with the anxiety, stress, and depression that may accompany the disorder. Involve family members and other potential caregivers in the educational program as much as possible.

Teach the patient and family about proper bronchial hygiene, including hydration, humidification of inspired air, postural drainage, and percussion techniques.

Emphasize the importance of infection control. Encourage the family to take measures to reduce the risk of infection, such as immunization against pneumococcal infection and influenza. If antibiotic therapy is prescribed, identify the correct methods for using the medications, and any danger or warning signs that should be reported to the health care provider.

Discuss the importance of maintaining weight at or just under the target weight. Nutrition plays an important role in successful coping with cystic fibrosis. Explain an appropriate diet and exercise regimen.

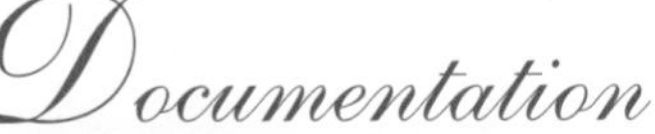

- Effectiveness of therapeutic measures
- Patient vital signs, weight, and skin, nail, and hair condition
- Patient intake and output, especially caloric intake

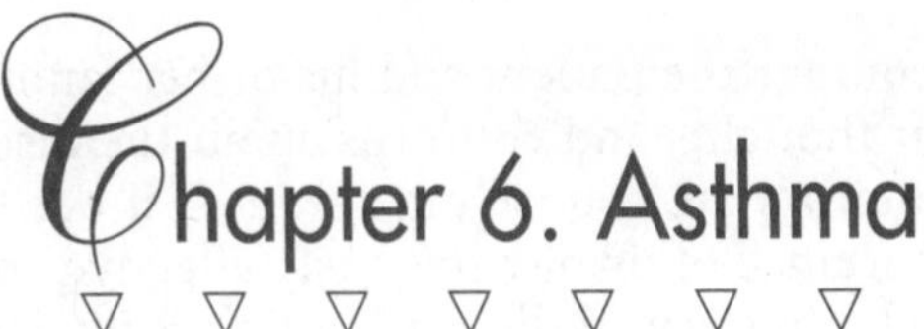

Chapter 6. Asthma

Introduction

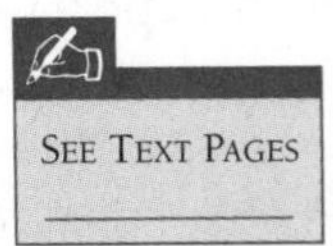

Asthma is characterized by hyperreactivity of the tracheobronchial tree to various stimuli and often associated with allergies. There are three types of asthma: extrinsic, or allergic, asthma; intrinsic, or idiopathic, asthma; and mixed asthma.

NURSING DIAGNOSES: IMPAIRED GAS EXCHANGE
INEFFECTIVE AIRWAY CLEARANCE
INEFFECTIVE BREATHING PATTERN

RELATED TO:

- *Increase in excessive mucus production, impaired ciliary movement, and chronic tissue hypoxia*

Nursing Interventions	Rationales
• Monitor respiratory status (for rate, effort, and breath sounds) and vital signs. Assess every 15 minutes to every several hours, depending on patient status.	• To identify impending respiratory failure
• Document baseline peak flow measurements, using a peak flow meter. Continue to document these measurements, after every aerosol treatment.	• To identify impending respiratory failure
• Elevate the patient's head and back (high Fowler's position), and arrange pillows to support the patient's respiratory efforts.	• To facilitate diaphragmatic excursion, keep the airway open, and alleviate discomfort during breathing
• Encourage the patient to expectorate secretions or perform suction, if needed.	• To clear blockage from respiratory passageways
• Document the color, consistency, and amount of secretions.	• To determine the effectiveness of treatment

Nursing Interventions *(Continued)*	Rationales *(Continued)*
• Teach the patient breathing exercises, such as incentive spirometry.	• To open alveolar passages and increase sputum expectoration
• Assist in performing chest physiotherapy, as needed.	• To help mobilize and eliminate lung secretions
• Encourage the patient to drink adequate amounts of fluid, at least 1,500 to 2,000 mL daily, unless the patient's fluid intake has been restricted.	• To help loosen secretions and compensate for fluid loss from secretion expectoration and elevated temperature

COLLABORATIVE MANAGEMENT

Interventions	Rationales
• Administer oxygen, as ordered.	• To prevent tissue hypoxia

NURSE ALERT:
Limit the fraction of inspired oxygen concentrations to those that achieve PaO_2 levels of 55 to 70 mm Hg. Higher PaO_2 levels may override the hypoxic drive needed to allow patients with COPD to breathe.

• Administer medications, as ordered: antibiotics, antipyretics, bronchodilators, expectorants, steroids.	• To resolve respiratory congestion, reduce fever, and reduce or prevent infection

OUTCOME:	EVALUATION CRITERIA:
• The patient will be able to breathe easily and effectively, sustain adequate ventilation, and maintain arterial blood gas values within normal ranges.	• Respirations are even and bilateral. • Edema of affected tissues is decreased. • Decreased pain or discomfort is reported.

NURSING DIAGNOSES: IMPAIRED GAS EXCHANGE *(CONTINUED)*

OUTCOME:
(Continued)

- The patient will be able to breathe easily and effectively, sustain adequate ventilation, and maintain arterial blood gas values within normal ranges. *(continued)*

EVALUATION CRITERIA:
(Continued)

- Uvula is located at midline.
- Pulse oximetry levels are adequate.

NURSING DIAGNOSIS: HIGH RISK FOR ACTIVITY INTOLERANCE

RELATED TO:

- *Dyspnea and fatigue*

Nursing Interventions	Rationales
• Plan patient care activities to take advantage of the patient's periods of energy.	• To avoid overtiring the patient

NURSE ALERT:
Generally, early morning and just after mealtime are not good times for patient care activities. In the morning, the patient will need to expend additional energy to clear nighttime secretions. After a meal, the patient will usually experience abdominal distention, putting a limit on diaphragmatic excursion, which increases breathing effort.

Nursing Interventions	Rationales
• Assist the patient in identifying his or her level of ability and point of fatigue.	• To encourage the patient to identify the need to get adequate rest
• Keep the patient's supplies, food, and possessions close at hand.	• To avoid increasing the patient's workload and to prevent additional exertion

COLLABORATIVE MANAGEMENT

Interventions	Rationales
• Consult with the physician and exercise physiologist to develop an exercise program for the patient.	• To increase the patient's stamina and work capacity

OUTCOME:	EVALUATION CRITERIA:
• The patient will be free from extended periods of extreme fatigue and will be able to perform activities of daily living with little effort or respiratory difficulty.	• Increased levels of activity are observed and reported. • The patient is able to complete activities of daily living.

NURSING DIAGNOSES: ANXIETY POWERLESSNESS

RELATED TO:

• *Uncertain outcome of the disorder, respiratory difficulties, and lack of information about the disorder, treatment plans, diagnostic tests, and procedures*

Nursing Interventions	Rationales
• Explain the condition to the patient and family members or other caregivers, using appropriate language for the patient's level of understanding.	• To ease unfamiliarity and discomfort and allow the patient some control over the situation
• Monitor the patient for signs of increasing distress, such as verbal or nonverbal communication.	• To prevent levels of anxiety and fear from becoming an additional burden on the patient's condition
• Maintain a calm, relaxed demeanor, and reassure the patient that his or her condition is being monitored at all times.	• To avoid additional anxiety concerning the staff's presence and attitude
• Encourage the patient to share his or her concerns, and respond to each as appropriate.	• To maintain open lines of communication

NURSING DIAGNOSES: ANXIETY *(CONTINUED)*

Nursing Interventions *(Continued)*	Rationales *(Continued)*
• Promote a quiet environment by reducing external stimulation.	• To limit the drain on the patient's resources—mental, emotional, and physical
• Plan care activities for times when the patient is feeling best able to handle the stress.	• To avoid unduly stressing the patient
• Encourage the patient to stop smoking and to ask other smokers to avoid smoking around him or her.	• To give the patient a means to exert some control over his or her condition
• Teach the patient about the role stress and emotions play in exacerbating infections and decreasing the body's ability to cope with illness.	• To promote the patient's control over his or her emotional well-being

COLLABORATIVE MANAGEMENT

Interventions	Rationales
• Administer medications, as ordered: sedatives.	• To decrease the patient's anxiety and fear
• Encourage the patient and family members to take advantage of counseling services and support groups, as appropriate.	• To develop effective coping skills

OUTCOME:	EVALUATION CRITERIA:
• The patient will appear calm and relaxed.	• Physical signs of distress, such as agitation, restlessness, and elevated respiratory rate are absent or decreased.
	• The patient reports that he or she is feeling more confident and relaxed.

NURSING DIAGNOSIS: KNOWLEDGE DEFICIT

RELATED TO:

- *Methods for delaying the progress of COPD, palliative measures, and maintaining optimum levels of health*

Nursing Interventions	Rationales
• Educate the patient about the pathophysiology of the disorder, prescribed medications and possible adverse effects, follow-up care requirements, and danger signs that should be reported to the health care provider.	• To increase the patient's understanding
• Include the patient's family and other caregivers in the educational program.	• To increase the likelihood that the patient will follow the self-care regimen

COLLABORATIVE MANAGEMENT

Interventions	Rationales
• Refer the patient, family, and other caregivers to the appropriate support agencies.	• To encourage understanding of the patient's condition
• Collaborate with other health care providers in stressing the importance of the health care regimen.	• To ensure understanding of the importance of the health care regimen

OUTCOME:	EVALUATION CRITERIA:
• The patient will demonstrate adequate knowledge about the disorder and self-care routines.	• The patient accurately describes the physical effects of the disorder. • The patient verbalizes an understanding of the use of medications, their adverse effects, and danger signs. • The patient complies with follow-up appointments and self-care regimen. • The patient seeks health care, if conditions indicate the need.

NURSING DIAGNOSIS: SOCIAL ISOLATION

RELATED TO:

- *Restrictions on activity or the withdrawal of friends and family members who are uncomfortable with the patient's disease*

Nursing Interventions	Rationales
• Discuss the changes in the patient's social activities that have been brought about by the disease. Identify any misconceptions the patient might have.	• To promote expression of the patient's concerns and questions
• Explain that although the disease does impose limitations on the patient's physical activity, reasonable exertion and exercise may actually improve the patient's condition. Caution the patient about starting a cycle of exercise avoidance, which leads to intolerance.	• To encourage the patient to remain as physically active as possible
• Educate the patient and his or her family and caregivers about the condition, its treatment requirements, and ways in which the patient can remain an active participant in many social activities.	• To increase patient and family understanding
• Encourage the patient to maintain and develop a network of friends and acquaintances with whom he or she can communicate frequently, in person, over the phone, by letter, or by computer.	• To develop additional outlets for social expression for the patient

COLLABORATIVE MANAGEMENT

Interventions	Rationales
• Identify support groups and other resources the patient can contact for information and advice, such as the American Lung Association.	• To promote the development of a support network
• Refer the patient to appropriate counseling to discuss issues related to social isolation and loneliness.	• To provide an additional outlet for the patient to express his or her feelings, fears, and concerns

OUTCOME:	EVALUATION CRITERIA:
• The patient will participate in social activities as appropriate for his or her condition.	• The patient expresses satisfaction with the social activities in which he or she is engaged. • The patient takes appropriate measures to promote his or her participation in social activities, such as engaging in an exercise program to build stamina.

Patient Teaching

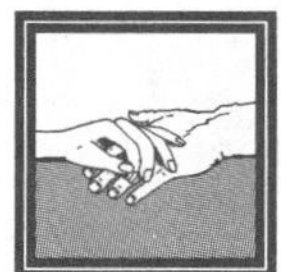

Stress that prevention of an asthma attack is always preferable to treating the patient for an attack. Help the patient to identify stressors and triggers that can bring on an attack. Common causes of asthma include:

- allergens, such as pollen, dust, and sulfites
- exercise or exertion
- cold air, especially a sudden change in air temperature
- drug reactions
- gastroesophageal reflux
- psychological or emotional stress

Encourage the patient to develop a plan for dealing with elements that may provoke an attack to prevent its occurrence. Help the patient to develop effective coping techniques if an attack should occur. Having a plan in place may help to reduce anxiety enough to alleviate an attack in the first place.

Demonstrate techniques for promoting effective breathing during an asthma attack. Instruct the patient to lean slightly forward and rest his or her elbows on a table, a counter, or his or her knees. The shoulders should be relaxed. As the patient inhales, he or she should lean forward slightly.

Instruct the patient about the proper use of bronchodilators and the use of various medications to control symptoms of the disorder.

Discuss the importance of maintaining weight at or just under the target weight. Extra weight increases breathing difficulty during attacks.

Encourage the patient to drink adequate amounts of fluid to help liquefy secretions and to replace fluid lost during an attack through sweating and hyperventilation.

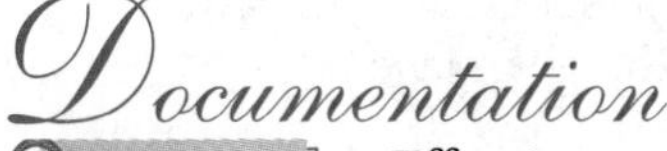

- Effectiveness of therapeutic measures
- Patient vital signs, weight, and skin, nail, and hair condition
- Patient intake and output, especially caloric intake

Suggested Readings

Corbin-West, A. L. "The Patient with Bronchospasm: Assessment, Triage and Teaching Adjuncts." *Journal of Emergency Nursing* 18, no. 6 (1992): 511–518.

Grossbach, I. "The COPD Patient in Acute Respiratory Failure." *Critical Care Nurse* 14, no. 6 (1994): 32–38.

SECTION III. INFECTIONS OF THE UPPER RESPIRATORY TRACT

Chapter 7. Tonsillitis and Pharyngitis

Introduction

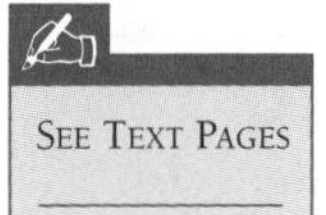
SEE TEXT PAGES ________

Tonsillitis is an inflammation of the tonsils and can be acute or chronic. Chronic tonsillitis is often the result of inadequately treated acute tonsillitis.

Pharyngitis, or acute sore throat, is almost always caused by infection. Occasionally, pain, when accompanied by inflammation or ulceration of the pharyngeal tissue, is caused by exposure to radiation or chemicals.

NURSING DIAGNOSIS: PAIN

RELATED TO:

- *Tonsillitis or pharyngitis*

Nursing Interventions	Rationales
• Assess the patient's level of discomfort, using a pain scale from 0 to 10.	• To help determine measures to take to adequately combat pain
• Monitor the patient's vital signs for indications of increased pain, such as rapid heart rate and elevated blood pressure.	• To assess for objective signs of worsening pain
• Address the patient's previous experiences with pain and how the patient coped with them.	• To encourage the use of previously successful coping mechanisms for controlling pain
• Teach the patient nonpharmacologic methods for controlling pain, such as meditation, guided imagery, and therapeutic touch.	• To relieve pain

NURSING DIAGNOSIS: PAIN *(CONTINUED)*

Nursing Interventions *(Continued)*	Rationales *(Continued)*
• Teach the patient about the pharmacologic interventions prescribed for him or her.	• To ensure that the patient knows when to ask for medication to prevent pain from becoming intolerable

COLLABORATIVE MANAGEMENT

Interventions	Rationales
• Consult with the pain management specialist about the best modes for treating the patient's pain (for example, when should pain be treated with medication or when should nonpharmacologic pain control methods be used).	• To provide better methods for controlling the pain and discomfort
• Administer medications, as ordered: analgesics, antipyretics, antitussives, topical anesthetics.	• To relieve pain, control fever, and reduce coughing

NURSE ALERT:
Sometimes patients are reluctant to give accurate reports of pain, causing health care providers to underestimate the dosage to prescribe or dispense.

OUTCOME:	EVALUATION CRITERIA:
• The patient will be free of pain.	• Pain is reported to be decreased or absent.
	• The pain scale rating is 4 or less.

NURSING DIAGNOSIS: HIGH RISK FOR INFECTION

RELATED TO:

- *Bacterial or viral invasion of tonsillar or pharyngeal tissue*

Nursing Interventions	Rationales
• Monitor vital signs for changes that indicate infection, such as elevated temperature and rapid heart rate.	• To prevent onset or worsening of infection
• Encourage the patient to drink fluids (1,500 to 2,000 mL daily), maintain adequate nutrition, and rest frequently.	• To prevent onset or worsening of infection
• Teach the patient basic infection control practices, such as hand washing and avoidance of other infected people.	• To minimize risk of contracting infection

COLLABORATIVE MANAGEMENT

Interventions	Rationales
• Administer medications, as ordered: antibiotics.	• To reduce or eliminate infection

NURSE ALERT:
Be careful to assess the patient for adverse reactions to drugs and food.

Interventions	Rationales
• Prepare the patient, if necessary, for surgery.	• To control infection

OUTCOME:

- The patient will be free of signs of infection.

EVALUATION CRITERIA:

- Vital signs are normal.
- Tissue is pinkish and unswollen.
- Pain is absent.

NURSING DIAGNOSIS: ALTERED ORAL MUCOUS MEMBRANE

RELATED TO:
- *Bacterial invasion of tonsillar or pharyngeal tissue*

Nursing Interventions	Rationales
• Encourage the patient to drink an adequate amount of fluid (1,500 to 2,000 mL daily).	• To keep mucosa hydrated and to compensate for elevated temperature
• Administer warm saline irrigation for the patient's throat.	• To ensure adequate tissue hydration

COLLABORATIVE MANAGEMENT

Interventions	Rationales
• Administer topical medications, as ordered: lozenges, topical anesthetics.	• To aid in tissue hydration

OUTCOME:	EVALUATION CRITERIA:
• The patient's mucous membrane will be adequately moist.	• Tissue is pinkish and unswollen.

NURSING DIAGNOSIS: IMPAIRED VERBAL COMMUNICATION

RELATED TO:
- *Laryngitis*

Nursing Interventions	Rationales
• Instruct the patient about the need to rest his or her voice.	• To provide an opportunity for healing and to decrease stress
• Apply an ice pack to the patient's anterior throat.	• To reduce swelling
• Encourage the patient to explore alternative methods of communication (for example, pad and pencil).	• To reduce the strain on healing tissues

COLLABORATIVE MANAGEMENT

Interventions	Rationales
• Administer topical medications as ordered: lozenges, over-the-counter sprays, topical anesthetics.	• To ease the effort in communicating

OUTCOME:	EVALUATION CRITERIA:
• The patient will be able to speak clearly without pain or discomfort.	• The patient demonstrates his or her ability to communicate without pain or discomfort.

NURSING DIAGNOSIS: INEFFECTIVE AIRWAY CLEARANCE

RELATED TO:

• *Inflammation and edema of tonsillar or pharyngeal tissue*

Nursing Interventions	Rationales
• Monitor respiratory status (for rate, effort, and breath sounds) and vital signs.	• To identify impending respiratory failure
• Elevate the patient's head and back (high Fowler's position), and arrange pillows to support the patient's respiratory efforts.	• To facilitate diaphragmatic excursion, keep the airway open, and alleviate discomfort during breathing
• Encourage the patient to expectorate secretions or perform suction, if needed.	• To clear secretions from respiratory passageways
• Teach the patient breathing exercises, such as incentive spirometry.	• To open alveolar passages and increase sputum expectoration
• Assist in performing chest physiotherapy, as needed.	• To help mobilize and eliminate lung secretions
• Encourage the patient to drink adequate amounts of fluid (1,500 to 2,000 mL daily).	• To help loosen secretions and to compensate for fluid loss from secretion expectoration and elevated temperature

NURSING DIAGNOSIS: INEFFECTIVE AIRWAY CLEARANCE

(CONTINUED)

Nursing Interventions *(Continued)*	Rationales *(Continued)*
• Apply an ice pack to the patient's throat, if appropriate.	• To reduce swelling

COLLABORATIVE MANAGEMENT

Interventions	Rationales
• Administer medications, as ordered: antibiotics, antipyretics, bronchodilators.	• To resolve respiratory congestion, control fever, and reduce or prevent infection
• Consult the respiratory therapist for information about chest physiotherapy.	• To ensure maximum benefit from therapy
• Assist with surgical incision and drainage procedures, if ordered.	• To maintain a patent airway

OUTCOME:	EVALUATION CRITERIA:
• The patient will be able to breathe easily and effectively, sustain adequate ventilation, and maintain arterial blood gas values within normal ranges.	• Respirations are even and bilateral. • Edema of affected tissues is decreased. • Pain or discomfort is decreased. • Uvula is located at midline. • Arterial blood gas values are within normal limits.

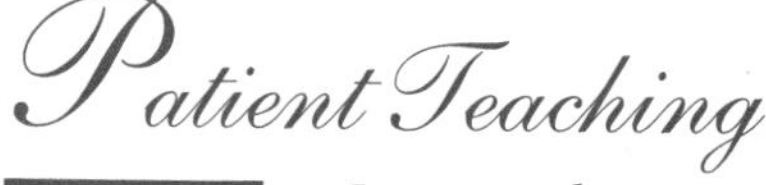

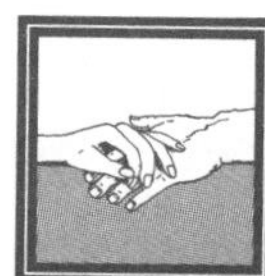

Instruct the patient to maintain adequate bed rest and, if appropriate, voice rest to promote healing.

Encourage the patient to maintain adequate fluid and food intake to facilitate the healing process. It may be necessary to experiment with different nutrition plans before settling on one that provides adequate nutrition.

Advise the patient about self-care routines that can prevent future occurrences or that are necessary after surgery. Stress the importance of completing the full course of antibiotic therapy to resolve any infection.

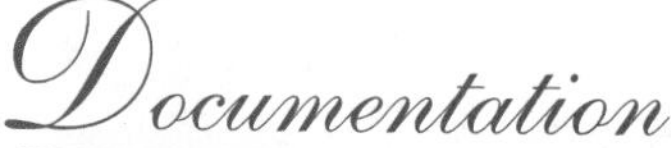

- Respiratory status, especially in acute presentations
- Effectiveness of medications administered and other interventions
- Response to self-care regimen instruction

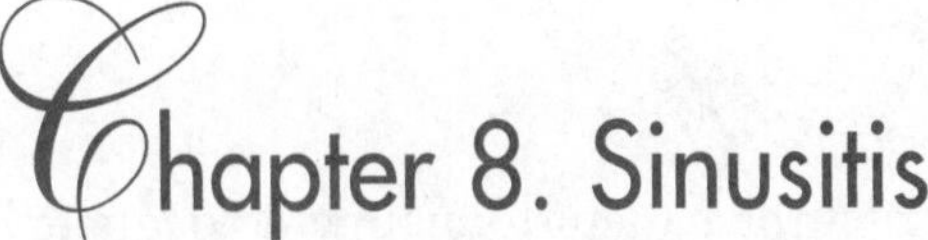

Chapter 8. Sinusitis

Introduction

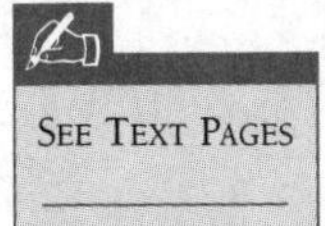

Sinusitis is inflammation of the sinuses and can be classified as acute or chronic. Many patients who suffer from acute sinusitis have recently had an upper respiratory tract viral infection. A patient with chronic sinusitis may find that the symptoms occur in response to allergies or because of some physical defect, such as a deviated septum.

NURSING DIAGNOSIS: PAIN

RELATED TO:

- *Inflammation of sinus tissue and accompanying pressure*

Nursing Interventions	Rationales
• Assess the patient's level of discomfort, using a pain scale from 0 to 10.	• To help determine measures to take to adequately combat pain
• Monitor vital signs for indications of increased pain, such as rapid heart rate and elevated blood pressure.	• To assess for objective signs of worsening pain
• Address the patient's previous experiences with pain and how the patient coped with them.	• To encourage the use of previously successful coping mechanisms for controlling pain
• Teach the patient nonpharmacologic methods for controlling pain, such as meditation, guided imagery, and therapeutic touch.	• To relieve pain
• Teach the patient about the pharmacologic interventions prescribed for him or her.	• To ensure that the patient knows when to ask for medication to prevent the pain from becoming intolerable
• Apply warm packs to the patient's face.	• To relieve pain

Nursing Interventions *(Continued)*	Rationales *(Continued)*
• Teach the patient methods for promoting sinus drainage.	• To relieve pressure causing pain
• Use vaporizing equipment to raise room humidity.	• To promote sinus drainage and relieve pressure

COLLABORATIVE MANAGEMENT

Interventions	Rationales
• Consult with the pain management specialist about the best modes for treating the patient's pain (for example, when should pain be treated with medication and when should nonpharmacologic pain control methods be used).	• To provide better methods for controlling the pain and discomfort
• Evaluate sinus radiographs and computed tomography scan, as ordered.	• To determine which sinuses are affected
• Administer medications, as ordered: analgesics, decongestants.	• To relieve pain and pressure

NURSE ALERT:
Sometimes patients are reluctant to give accurate reports of pain, causing health care providers to underestimate the dosage to prescribe or dispense.

Interventions	Rationales
• Assist in direct needle puncture and aspiration, as ordered.	• To reduce pain

OUTCOME:	EVALUATION CRITERIA:
• The patient will be free of pain.	• Pain is reported to be decreased or absent.
	• The pain scale rating is 4 or less.

NURSING DIAGNOSIS: HIGH RISK FOR INFECTION

RELATED TO:

- *Bacterial invasion of sinus tissue*

Nursing Interventions	Rationales
• Monitor vital signs for changes that indicate infection, such as elevated temperature and rapid heart rate.	• To prevent onset or worsening of infection
• Encourage the patient to drink fluids (1,500 to 2,000 mL daily), maintain adequate nutrition, and rest frequently.	• To prevent onset or worsening of infection
• Teach the patient basic infection control practices, such as hand washing and avoidance of other infected people.	• To minimize risk of contracting infection

COLLABORATIVE MANAGEMENT

Interventions	Rationales
• Administer medications, as ordered: antibiotics.	• To reduce or eliminate infection

NURSE ALERT:
Be careful to assess the patient for adverse reactions to drugs and food.

Interventions	Rationales
• Prepare the patient, if necessary, for surgery.	• To control infection
• Collect fluid sample and send it to the laboratory for culture, as ordered.	• To determine the origin of the infection

OUTCOME:

- The patient will be free of signs of infection.

EVALUATION CRITERIA:

- Vital signs are normal.
- Drainage from sinuses is decreased.

NURSING DIAGNOSIS: KNOWLEDGE DEFICIT

RELATED TO:

- *Measures available for prevention of sinusitis and appropriate health care regimen*

Nursing Interventions	Rationales
• Explain medications, treatment plan, and diagnostic tests to the patient or caregiver.	• To ensure adequate understanding of the health care regimen
• Emphasize the need for the patient to follow the treatment recommendations and to notify the health care provider if the infection worsens or shows no signs of improvement within 3 to 5 days (elevated temperature for more than 1 week, continued purulent drainage).	• To ensure compliance with the health care regimen

COLLABORATIVE MANAGEMENT

Interventions	Rationales
• Collaborate with other health care providers in stressing the importance of complying with the health care regimen.	• To ensure understanding of the disorder and the necessary health care regimen

OUTCOME:	EVALUATION CRITERIA:
• The patient will demonstrate adequate knowledge about his or her disorder and appropriate self-care behaviors.	• The patient complies with the self-care regimen. • The patient demonstrates self-care techniques.

Patient Teaching

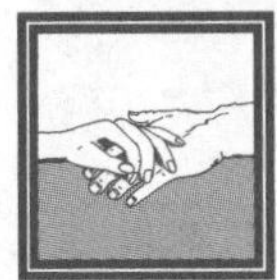

Instruct the patient in the proper use and adverse effects of the prescribed medications. Emphasize the importance of completing the full course of treatment and notifying the health care provider if the infection worsens or does not respond appropriately.

Demonstrate nonpharmacologic methods for easing discomfort, including the use of hot packs, room vaporizers, facial saunas, and hot showers for loosening congestion.

Documentation

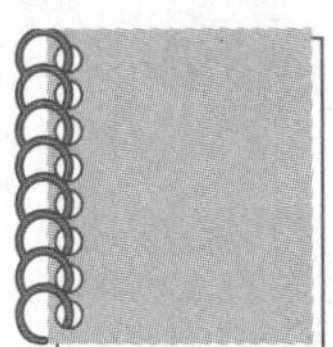

- Effectiveness of treatment and patient compliance with regimen
- If radiographs were ordered at the onset of treatment, follow-up radiographs may be required to demonstrate the resolution of infection.

Nursing Research

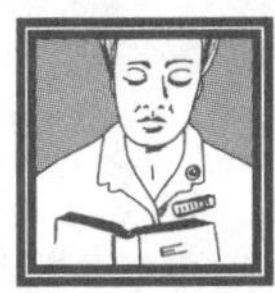

Most clinicians find that symptoms of sinusitis are relieved by a short course of topical or systemic decongestants. It is also possible that such a treatment accelerates infection resolution by promoting drainage.

Gantz, Nelson M., and Alan J. Sogg. "An Update on Sinusitis." *Patient Care* (April 1992): 141–163.

Suggested Readings

Clendenen, K. "A Tornado by the Tail: The Importance of Initial Assessment." *Today's OR Nurse* 13, no. 12 (1991): 25–28.

Schwartz, R. H. "Tonsillectomy Today—Who Needs It?" *Patient Care* 26 (January 1992): 173–194.

SECTION IV. INFECTIONS OF THE LOWER RESPIRATORY TRACT

Chapter 9. Pneumonia

Introduction

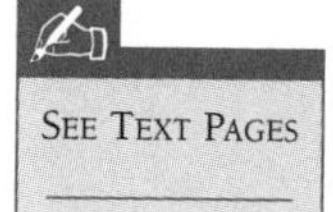
SEE TEXT PAGES ______

Pneumonia is a severe inflammation of the pulmonary tissue. One of the ways in which pneumonia can be classified is according to the area of the lung that is affected. Bronchopneumonia involves patchy areas in several lobules of the lung. Interstitial pneumonia affects the wall around the bronchioles and alveoli. Lobar pneumonia affects a large portion or an entire lobe of a lung.

NURSING DIAGNOSIS: PAIN

RELATED TO:

- *Pleuritic changes that accompany pneumonia*

Nursing Interventions	Rationales
• Assess the patient's level of discomfort, using a pain scale from 0 to 10.	• To help determine measures to take to adequately combat pain
• Monitor vital signs for indications of increased pain, such as rapid heart rate and elevated blood pressure.	• To assess for objective signs of worsening pain
• Address the patient's previous experiences with pain and how the patient coped with them.	• To encourage the use of previously successful coping mechanisms for controlling pain
• Teach the patient nonpharmacologic methods for controlling pain, such as meditation, guided imagery, and therapeutic touch.	• To relieve pain
• Teach the patient about the pharmacologic interventions prescribed for him or her.	• To ensure that the patient knows when to ask for medication to prevent pain from becoming intolerable

NURSING DIAGNOSIS: PAIN *(CONTINUED)*

COLLABORATIVE MANAGEMENT

Interventions	Rationales
• Consult with the pain management specialist about the best modes for treating the patient's pain (for example, when should pain be treated with medication or when should nonpharmacologic pain control methods be used).	• To provide better methods for controlling the pain and discomfort
• Administer medications, as ordered: analgesics, antibiotics, sedatives.	• To relieve pain and reduce infection

NURSE ALERT:
Sometimes patients are reluctant to give accurate reports of pain, causing health care providers to underestimate the dosage to prescribe or dispense.

NURSE ALERT:
Be careful to assess the patient for adverse reactions to drugs and food.

Interventions	Rationales
• Assist in administering chest physiotherapy, as ordered.	• To help mobilize and eliminate lung secretions and lessen discomfort

OUTCOME:	EVALUATION CRITERIA:
• The patient will be free of pain.	• Pain is reported to be decreased or absent.
	• The pain scale rating is 4 or less.

NURSING DIAGNOSIS: HIGH RISK FOR INFECTION

RELATED TO:

- *Weakened immune system caused by pneumonia*

Nursing Interventions	Rationales
• Monitor vital signs for changes that indicate infection, such as elevated temperature and rapid heart rate.	• To prevent onset or worsening of infection
• Encourage the patient to drink fluids (1,500 to 2,000 mL daily), maintain adequate nutrition, and rest frequently.	• To prevent onset or worsening of infection
• Teach the patient basic infection control practices, such as hand washing and avoidance of other infected people.	• To minimize the risk of contracting infection
• Follow strict hygiene routines when caring for the patient, especially when suctioning.	• To minimize the risk of contracting infection

COLLABORATIVE MANAGEMENT

Interventions	Rationales
• Administer medications, as ordered: antibiotics, antipyretics, bronchodilators, inhaled steroids.	• To reduce or eliminate infection and control fever
• Examine sputum and blood cultures.	• To determine causative agent
• Consult the respiratory therapist for information about inhaled medications.	• To ensure the proper use of medications
• Consult the pharmacist for information about the adverse effects of medications ordered, especially their interactions with one another and with food ordered for the patient.	• To prevent adverse drug reactions

NURSING DIAGNOSIS: HIGH RISK FOR INFECTION *(CONTINUED)*

OUTCOME:	EVALUATION CRITERIA:
• The patient will be free of signs of infection.	• Vital signs are normal. • Tissue is pinkish and unswollen.

NURSING DIAGNOSIS: FLUID VOLUME DEFICIT

RELATED TO:

- *Increased metabolic demands from fever, the disease process, and diaphoresis*

Nursing Interventions	Rationales
• Monitor the patient's fluid intake and output.	• To determine patterns of intake and output to more easily identify variations
• Maintain patency of I.V. lines and drainage tubes.	• To assure adequate fluid intake and output
• Encourage the patient to drink adequate amounts of fluid, at least 1,500 to 2,000 mL daily, unless the patient's fluid intake has been restricted.	• To compensate for fluid loss
• Provide cooling measures such as cooling blankets and sponge baths.	• To reduce effects of fever
• Assess for other signs of fluid volume deficit, such as altered mental status, increased anxiety, increased heart rate, jugular vein distention, poor skin turgor, dehydrated mucous membranes, and hypotension.	• To assure early detection of fluid volume deficit

COLLABORATIVE MANAGEMENT

Interventions	Rationales
• Assess laboratory values for central venous pressure status, complete blood count, creatinine and electrolyte levels, and baseline hematocrit and hemoglobin.	• To assure early detection of fluid volume deficit
• Prepare the patient for a transfusion, if ordered.	• To alleviate fluid volume deficit
• Administer a blood or fluid transfusion, as ordered.	• To alleviate fluid volume deficit
• Administer medications, as ordered: antipyretics.	• To control fever

OUTCOME:

- The patient will experience adequate fluid volume.

EVALUATION CRITERIA:

- Urine output is normal (>30 mL/hr.).
- Serum electrolyte levels are within normal limits.
- Arterial blood gas values are within normal limits.
- Central venous pressure measurements are within normal limits.
- Vital signs are stable.

NURSING DIAGNOSIS: ANXIETY

RELATED TO:

- *Effects of pneumonia, the course and outcome of the disorder, and a lack of knowledge about the treatment and health care regimen*

Nursing Interventions	Rationales
• Assess the patient for verbal and nonverbal signs of anxiety.	• To identify trends indicating worsening anxiety

NURSING DIAGNOSIS: ANXIETY *(CONTINUED)*

Nursing Interventions *(Continued)*	Rationales *(Continued)*
• Explain the physical effects that pneumonia will cause, such as bouts of dyspnea and production of bloody sputum, and emphasize that they are common.	• To alleviate fear and embarrassment
• Explain care routines and the tests and treatments the patient will undergo.	• To reduce the lack of knowledge about pneumonia and help the patient prepare for upcoming events, thus giving the patient a feeling of greater control

COLLABORATIVE MANAGEMENT

Interventions	Rationales
• Involve the family and appropriate social and spiritual caregivers in the patient's efforts to reduce anxiety.	• To lessen anxiety

OUTCOME:	EVALUATION CRITERIA:
• The patient will experience reduced anxiety related to his or her disorder.	• The patient expresses an understanding of the course and treatment of pneumonia.

NURSING DIAGNOSIS: INEFFECTIVE AIRWAY CLEARANCE

RELATED TO:

- *Increased secretions in the alveoli and inflammation of respiratory passageways*

Nursing Interventions	Rationales
• Monitor respiratory status (for rate, effort, and breath sounds) and vital signs.	• To identify impending respiratory failure
• Elevate the patient's head and back (high Fowler's position), and arrange pillows to support the patient's respiratory efforts.	• To facilitate diaphragmatic excursion, keep the airway open, and alleviate discomfort during breathing

Nursing Interventions *(Continued)*	Rationales *(Continued)*
• Encourage the patient to expectorate secretions or perform suction, if needed.	• To clear secretions from respiratory passageways
• Teach the patient breathing exercises, such as incentive spirometry.	• To open alveolar passages and increase sputum expectoration
• Assist in performing chest physiotherapy, as needed.	• To help mobilize and eliminate lung secretions
• Encourage the patient to drink adequate amounts of fluid (1,500 to 2,000 mL daily).	• To help loosen secretions and compensate for fluid loss from secretion expectoration and elevated temperature

COLLABORATIVE MANAGEMENT

Interventions	Rationales
• Administer medications, as ordered: antibiotics, antipyretics, bronchodilators.	• To resolve respiratory congestion, control fever, and reduce or prevent infection
• Consult the respiratory therapist for information about chest physiotherapy.	• To ensure the maximum benefit from therapy
• Assist with surgical incision and drainage procedures, if ordered.	• To maintain a patent airway

OUTCOME:	EVALUATION CRITERIA:
• The patient will be able to breathe easily and effectively, sustain adequate ventilation, and maintain arterial blood gas values within normal ranges.	• Respirations are even and bilateral. • Edema of affected tissues is decreased. • Pain or discomfort is reported to be decreased. • Uvula is located at midline.

NURSING DIAGNOSIS: IMPAIRED GAS EXCHANGE

RELATED TO:
- *Tissue consolidation*

Nursing Interventions	Rationales
• Monitor arterial blood gas values, especially $Paco_2$, because an elevated $Paco_2$ value is the first sign of impending respiratory failure.	• To assess the status of oxygenation
• Monitor for signs of impending respiratory failure.	• To allow for medical intervention at the earliest point possible
• Administer oxygen, as ordered.	• To prevent tissue hypoxia
• Alleviate the patient's anxiety and reduce metabolic demands.	• To help control tissue demand for oxygen

COLLABORATIVE MANAGEMENT

Interventions	Rationales
• Assist with immediate interventions, such as intubation and mechanical ventilation, especially if respiratory failure or tissue hypoxia is present.	• To prevent respiratory failure
• Consult with the respiratory therapist to determine the most appropriate oxygen-flow device for the patient.	• To ensure an adequate supply of oxygen
• Administer medications, as ordered: antianxiety agents, sedatives.	• To reduce metabolic demands for oxygen
• Schedule chest radiographs and sputum cultures, as ordered.	• To monitor respiratory status

NURSING DIAGNOSIS: IMPAIRED GAS EXCHANGE *(CONTINUED)*

OUTCOME:

- The patient will regain and maintain adequate ventilation.

EVALUATION CRITERIA:

- Arterial blood gas values are within normal ranges.
- There is no evidence of cyanosis.
- Breathing is easy and relaxed, as indicated by physical signs and the patient's assessment of respiratory effort.

NURSING DIAGNOSIS: INEFFECTIVE BREATHING PATTERN

RELATED TO:

- *Increasing respiratory difficulties and the patient's perception that he or she "can't get a good breath"*

Nursing Interventions	Rationales
• Assist with postural drainage (every 2 hours).	• To drain secretions and keep airways open
• Encourage the patient to cough productively and clear secretions, using incentive spirometry, if appropriate.	• To clear respiratory passageways and ease breathing patterns
• Elevate the patient's head and support the chest and back.	• To aid respiration by allowing for diaphragmatic excursion
• Teach the patient effective breathing techniques, such as pursed-lip and diaphragmatic breathing.	• To increase alveolar expansion and mucus expectoration

NURSING DIAGNOSIS: INEFFECTIVE BREATHING PATTERN
(CONTINUED)

COLLABORATIVE MANAGEMENT

Interventions	Rationales
• Consult with the respiratory therapist about the most effective plan for breathing exercises and chest physiotherapy.	• To aid respiration

OUTCOME:	EVALUATION CRITERIA:
• The patient will maintain a regular, efficient breathing pattern.	• Breathing pattern is normal. • There is no evidence of cyanosis.

DRAINAGE POSITIONS FOR VARIOUS LUNG AREAS

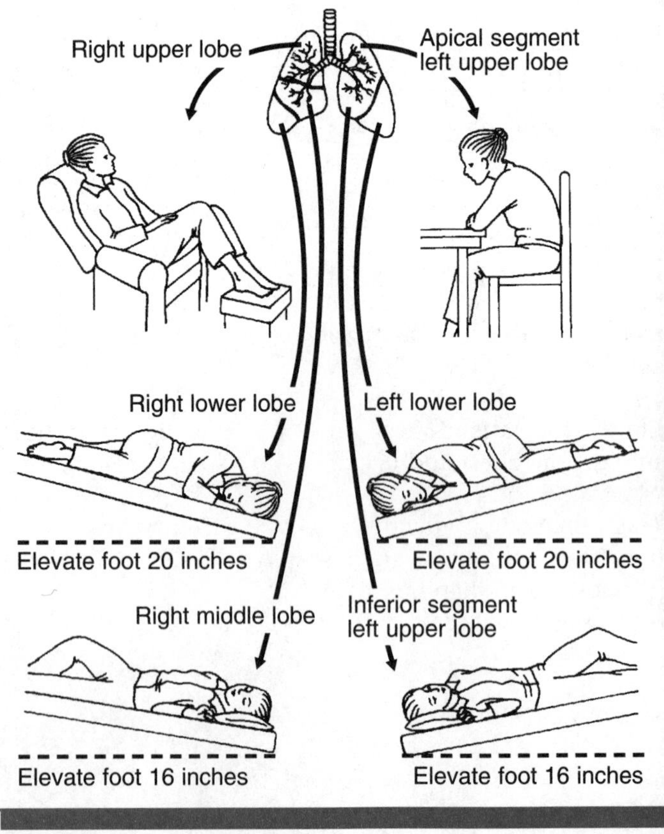

Right upper lobe
Apical segment left upper lobe
Right lower lobe
Elevate foot 20 inches
Left lower lobe
Elevate foot 20 inches
Right middle lobe
Elevate foot 16 inches
Inferior segment left upper lobe
Elevate foot 16 inches

NURSING DIAGNOSIS: HIGH RISK FOR ASPIRATION

RELATED TO:

- *Patient's inability to effectively clear increased secretions*

Nursing Interventions	Rationales
• Assess the patient's respiratory status frequently.	• To identify signs of aspiration of secretions
• Monitor vital signs for indications of infection caused by aspiration of purulent secretions. Such an infection may develop into bronchiectasis.	• To identify infection and begin treatment
• Assist the patient to maintain a comfortable position, with the head of the bed elevated, unless contraindicated.	• To reduce the risk of aspiration and facilitate drainage
• Teach the patient effective coughing techniques and assist him or her to expectorate secretions.	• To promote the removeal of secretions
• If the patient is entubated, monitor him or her carefully for signs of aspiration. Suction airway, as needed.	• To reduce the risk of aspiration and identify signs of respiratory distress

COLLABORATIVE MANAGEMENT

Interventions	Rationales
• Consult with speech pathologists to schedule an evaluation of the patient's swallowing abilities.	• To rule out underlying potential physical causes of aspiration
• Administer antibiotics, as ordered.	• To resolve any infections caused by aspiration of secretions, thereby reducing the production of additional secretions which often accompanies infection

NURSING DIAGNOSIS: HIGH RISK FOR ASPIRATION *(CONTINUED)*

OUTCOME:

- The patient will not aspirate pulmonary secretions.

EVALUATION CRITERIA:

- Respiratory status is normal.
- The patient can effectively clear his or her own secretions.
- Signs of infection are absent.

Patient Teaching

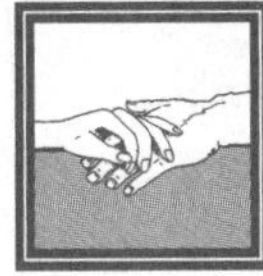

Inform the patient about the normal course of treatment and tests, and reassure him or her that breathing should be easier within a few days after treatment has begun.

Emphasize the need to expectorate lung secretions. Remind the patient that this will make breathing easier and help to alleviate the need for additional measures, such as oxygen therapy.

Encourage the patient to use good pulmonary hygiene techniques, such as avoiding smoke and other irritants.

Inform the patient about the use of prescribed medications, such as bronchodilators and antibiotics. Include information about adverse reactions, drug interactions, and the importance of completing the full course of therapy.

Teach the patient effective breathing techniques, such as pursed-lip breathing, diaphragmatic breathing, and incentive spirometry.

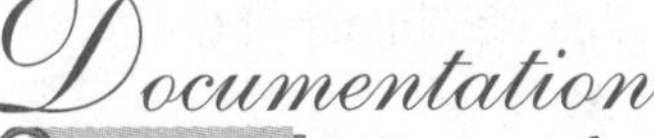

Documentation

- Patient's level of activity and respiratory effort
- Arterial blood gas values
- Patient response to medication
- Patient compliance with health care regimen

Chapter 10: Tuberculosis

▽ ▽ ▽ ▽ ▽ ▽ ▽

Introduction

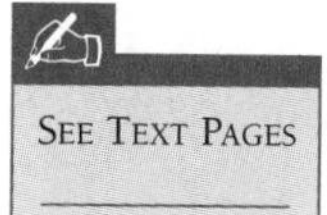

Tuberculosis is an infectious disease that is caused by exposure to *Mycobacterium tuberculosis* or *Mycobacterium bovis* by way of the respiratory tract, the gastrointestinal tract, or an open wound. Patients who suffer from this disease exhibit signs and symptoms of pneumonia or chronic bronchitis. The diagnosis of tuberculosis is confirmed when positive identification of tuberculosis bacterium cultures is made.

NURSING DIAGNOSIS: INEFFECTIVE AIRWAY CLEARANCE

RELATED TO:

- *Increased secretions in the alveoli and inflammation of respiratory passageways*

Nursing Interventions	Rationales
• Monitor respiratory status (for rate, effort, and breath sounds) and vital signs.	• To identify impending respiratory failure
• Elevate the patient's head and back (high Fowler's position), and arrange pillows to support the patient's respiratory efforts.	• To facilitate diaphragmatic excursion, keep the airway open, and alleviate discomfort during breathing
• Encourage the patient to expectorate secretions or perform suction, if needed.	• To clear secretions from respiratory passageways
• Teach the patient breathing exercises, such as incentive spirometry or pursed-lip breathing.	• To open alveolar passages and increase sputum expectoration
• Assist in performing chest physiotherapy, as needed.	• To help mobilize and eliminate lung secretions
• Encourage the patient to drink adequate amounts of fluid (1,500 to 2,000 mL daily).	• To help loosen secretions and compensate for fluid loss from secretion expectoration and elevated temperature

NURSING DIAGNOSIS: INEFFECTIVE AIRWAY CLEARANCE (CONTINUED)

COLLABORATIVE MANAGEMENT

Interventions	Rationales
• Administer medications, as ordered: antibiotics, antipyretics, bronchodilators.	• To resolve respiratory congestion, control fever, and reduce or prevent infection

NURSE ALERT:
Be careful to assess the patient for adverse reactions to drugs and food.

Interventions	Rationales
• Consult the respiratory therapist for information about chest physiotherapy.	• To ensure the maximum benefit from therapy
• Assist with surgical incision and drainage procedures, if ordered.	• To maintain a patent airway
• Follow your facility's protocol for patient isolation until infectious disease clinicians determine that the risk is over.	• To prevent the spread of infection

OUTCOME:

- The patient will be able to breathe easily and effectively, sustain adequate ventilation, and maintain arterial blood gas values within normal ranges.

EVALUATION CRITERIA:

- Respirations are even and bilateral.
- Edema of affected tissues is decreased.
- Pain or discomfort is reported to be decreased.
- Uvula is located at midline.
- Arterial blood gas values are within normal limits.

NURSING DIAGNOSIS: IMPAIRED GAS EXCHANGE

RELATED TO:

- *Tissue consolidation and decreased area available for gas exchange*

Nursing Interventions	Rationales
• Monitor arterial blood gas values and respiratory status.	• To assess the status of oxygenation
• Monitor for signs of impending respiratory failure, such as tachypnea, restlessness, cyanosis, confusion, and accessory muscle use.	• To allow for earliest possible medical intervention
• Administer oxygen, as ordered.	• To promote adequate tissue oxygenation

COLLABORATIVE MANAGEMENT

Interventions	Rationales
• Assist with bronchoscopy, if ordered.	• To remove persistent secretions
• Collect sputum samples, as ordered.	• To monitor the patient's condition and the effectiveness of treatment

OUTCOME:	EVALUATION CRITERIA:
• The patient will regain and maintain adequate ventilation.	• Arterial blood gas values are within normal ranges. • There is no evidence of cyanosis. • Breathing is easy and relaxed.

NURSING DIAGNOSIS: SOCIAL ISOLATION

RELATED TO:

- *Infection with a contagious disease*

Nursing Interventions	Rationales
• Educate the patient about the risks associated with the disease, and assist in developing a plan for getting the most out of limited social visits.	• To ease feelings of isolation
• Encourage the patient to use alternate means of communication, such as telephone conversations and letter writing.	• To maintain social contact while reducing the risk of contagion
• Urge the patient to express his or her concerns and feelings. Reassure the patient that the period of isolation will end and normal levels of social contact can be resumed.	• To ease feelings of isolation

COLLABORATIVE MANAGEMENT

Interventions	Rationales
• Refer the patient, family, and other caregivers to appropriate support groups and social agencies.	• To learn ways of coping with social isolation

OUTCOME:	EVALUATION CRITERIA:
• The patient will initiate social contact within the limits imposed by the disease.	• Independent socialization activities are conducted. • Effective coping skills for dealing with isolation are verbalized and used.

NURSING DIAGNOSIS: KNOWLEDGE DEFICIT

RELATED TO:

- *Course of the disorder, treatment plans, and self-care routines*

Nursing Interventions	Rationales
• Educate the patient about the pathophysiology of the disease, prescribed medications and their adverse effects, follow-up care requirements, and danger signs that should be reported to the health care provider.	• To increase understanding of the disease
• Include the patient's family and other caregivers in the educational program.	• To increase the likelihood that the self-care regimen is followed
• Discuss with the patient the stigma associated with a having a contagious disease.	• To increase understanding of others' reactions

COLLABORATIVE MANAGEMENT

Interventions	Rationales
• Refer the patient, family, and other caregivers to the appropriate support agencies.	• To encourage understanding of the patient's disease
• Collaborate with other health care providers in stressing the importance of the health care regimen.	• To ensure understanding of the importance of the health care regimen

OUTCOME:	EVALUATION CRITERIA:
• The patient will demonstrate adequate knowledge about the disease and self-care routines.	• The patient accurately describes the physical effects of the disease. • The patient verbalizes an understanding of the use of medications, their adverse effects, and danger signs. • The patient complies with follow-up appointments and the self-care regimen.

NURSING DIAGNOSIS: KNOWLEDGE DEFICIT *(CONTINUED)*

OUTCOME:
(Continued)

- The patient will demonstrate adequate knowledge about the disease and self-care routines. *(continued)*

EVALUATION CRITERIA:
(Continued)

- The patient seeks health care if conditions indicate the need.

NURSING DIAGNOSIS: FLUID VOLUME DEFICIT

RELATED TO:

- *Increased metabolic demands and inadequate fluid intake*

Nursing Interventions	Rationales
• Monitor the patient's fluid intake and output.	• To determine patterns of intake and output to more easily identify variations
• Maintain the patency of I.V. lines and drainage tubes.	• To assure adequate fluid intake and output
• Encourage the patient to drink adequate amounts of fluid, at least 1,500 to 2,000 mL daily, unless the patient's fluid intake has been restricted.	• To compensate for fluid loss
• Assess for other signs of fluid volume deficit, such as altered mental status, increased anxiety, increased heart rate, jugular vein distention, poor skin turgor, dehydrated mucous membranes, and hypotension.	• To assure early detection of fluid volume deficit

COLLABORATIVE MANAGEMENT

Interventions	Rationales
• Assess laboratory values for central venous pressure status, complete blood count, creatinine and electrolyte levels, and baseline hematocrit and hemoglobin.	• To assure early detection of fluid volume deficit

COLLABORATIVE MANAGEMENT *(CONTINUED)*

Interventions *(Continued)*	Rationales *(Continued)*
• Prepare the patient for a transfusion, if ordered.	• To alleviate fluid volume deficit
• Administer a blood or fluid transfusion, as ordered.	• To alleviate fluid volume deficit

OUTCOME:	EVALUATION CRITERIA:
• The patient will experience adequate fluid volume.	• Urine output is normal (>30 mL/hr.). • Serum electrolyte levels are within normal limits. • Arterial blood gas values are within normal limits. • Central venous pressure measurements are within normal limits. • Vital signs are stable.

Patient Teaching

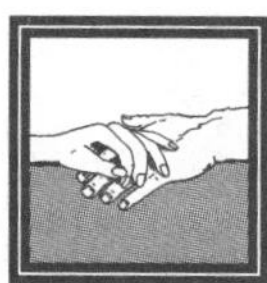

Explain the nature of the disease and the process of infection. Reinforce precautions for avoiding contamination (use of air masks, covering the mouth and nose when coughing, limiting social contact).

Instruct the patient in the necessary self-care and follow-up measures. Remind the patient of the importance of completing the full course of antibiotic therapy to ensure resolution of the infection. This is especially important in cases of tuberculosis, where treatment may be prescribed for many months.

Documentation

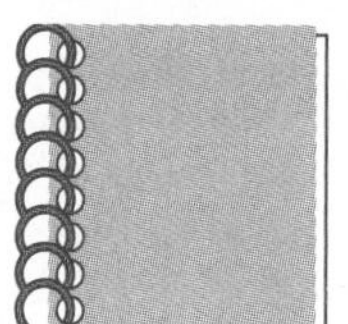

- Time and circumstances of acid-fast bacterium isolation, if ordered
- Contact with public health officials
- Results of sputum testing
- Patient compliance with therapeutic regimen

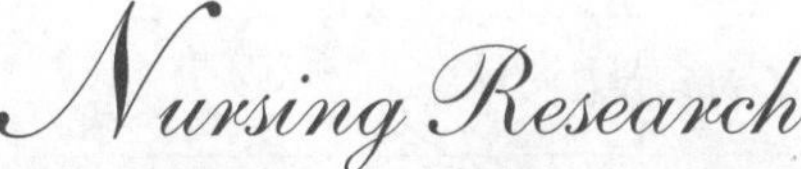

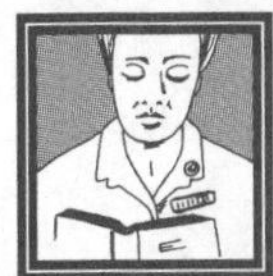

The use of a numeric rating system to be used in emergency departments is being investigated at some hospitals. It would identify during triage those patients with risk factors and symptoms indicative of tuberculosis. In this way, the need for immediate isolation and diagnostic procedures is more clearly indicated. Research has shown that earlier diagnosis and treatment improve the patient's chance for survival.

Lewis, R. J., G. Sokolove, D. Mackey, J. Krawczyk, and J. Wiles. "A Triage Procedure for the Detection and Isolation of Patients at High Risk for Active Pulmonary Tuberculosis." *Academy of Emergency Medicine* 1, no. 2 (1994): A29.

Chapter 11: Lung Abscess

Introduction

SEE TEXT PAGES

Lung abscess is a localized infection of the lung parenchyma in which there is an accumulation of pus and destruction of lung tissue. It is usually caused by anaerobic bacteria. It is also called necrotizing pneumonia or pulmonary abscess. Patients who suffer from chronic lung abscess may develop bronchiectasis.

NURSING DIAGNOSIS: PAIN

RELATED TO:

- *Inflammation of pulmonary tissue*

Nursing Interventions	Rationales
• Assess the patient's level of discomfort, using a pain scale from 0 to 10.	• To help determine measures to take to adequately combat the pain
• Monitor vital signs for indications of increased pain, such as rapid heart rate and elevated blood pressure.	• To assess for objective signs of worsening pain
• Address the patient's previous experiences with pain and how the patient coped with them.	• To encourage the use of previously successful coping mechanisms for controlling pain
• Teach the patient nonpharmacologic methods for controlling pain, such as meditation, guided imagery, and therapeutic touch.	• To relieve pain
• Teach the patient about the pharmacologic interventions prescribed for him or her.	• To ensure that the patient knows when to ask for medication to prevent pain from becoming intolerable

NURSING DIAGNOSIS: PAIN *(CONTINUED)*

COLLABORATIVE MANAGEMENT

Interventions	Rationales
• Consult with the pain management specialist about the best modes for treating the patient's pain (for example, when should pain be treated with medication or when should nonpharmacologic pain control methods be used).	• To provide better methods for controlling the pain and discomfort
• Administer medications, as ordered: analgesics, antipyretics, antitussives, topical anesthetics.	• To relieve pain, control fever, and reduce coughing

NURSE ALERT:
Sometimes patients are reluctant to give accurate reports of pain, causing health care providers to underestimate the dosage to prescribe or dispense.

OUTCOME:	EVALUATION CRITERIA:
• The patient will have minimal or no pain.	• Pain is reported to be decreased or absent. • The pain scale rating is 4 or less.

NURSING DIAGNOSIS: HIGH RISK FOR INFECTION

RELATED TO:

- *Infectious agent (usually bacteria)*

Nursing Interventions	Rationales
• Monitor vital signs for changes that indicate infection, such as elevated temperature and rapid heart rate.	• To prevent onset or worsening of infection
• Encourage the patient to drink fluids (1,500 to 2,000 mL daily), maintain adequate nutrition, and rest frequently.	• To prevent onset or worsening of infection
• Teach the patient basic infection control practices, such as hand washing and avoidance of other infected people.	• To minimize the risk of contracting infection
• Assess laboratory test results (white blood cell count, blood or sputum cultures).	• To identify the occurrence or worsening of infection
• Assist the patient with the postural drainage routine several times daily.	• To promote the removal of abscess secretions

NURSE ALERT:
Postural drainage must be done with extreme care to avoid spreading infection to healthy areas of the lung.

COLLABORATIVE MANAGEMENT

Interventions	Rationales
• Administer medications, as ordered: antibiotics.	• To reduce or eliminate infection

NURSING DIAGNOSIS: HIGH RISK FOR INFECTION *(CONTINUED)*

COLLABORATIVE MANAGEMENT

Interventions *(Continued)*	Rationales *(Continued)*
• Prepare the patient, if necessary, for surgery.	• To control infection
• Assist with bronchoscopy, if ordered.	• To use cultures in the diagnosis or as a therapeutic measure

OUTCOME:	EVALUATION CRITERIA:
• The patient will be free of signs of infection.	• Vital signs are normal. • Sputum cultures are negative. • White blood cell count is normal.

Patient Teaching

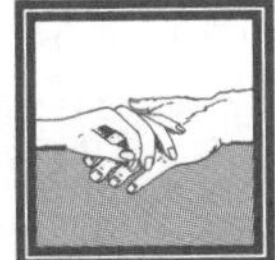

Instruct the patient about the need to resolve the infection to prevent worsening of the condition into bronchiectasis.

Documentation

- Patient tolerance of therapeutic regimen
- Vital signs and laboratory test results

Suggested Readings

Boutotte, J. "TB—The Second Time Around." *Nursing93* 23, no. 5 (1993): 42–49.

Stiesmeyer, J. K. "A Four Step Approach to Pulmonary Assessment." *American Journal of Nursing* 93, no. 8 (1993): 22–28.

SECTION V. RESPIRATORY NEOPLASMS

Chapter 12. Lung Cancer

Introduction

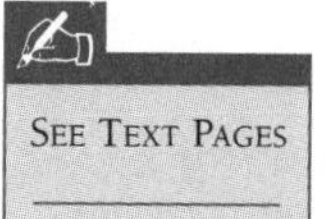
SEE TEXT PAGES ______

Lung cancer, one of the most common cancers, is largely preventable. It is typically classified as small-cell carcinoma or non–small-cell carcinoma. Non–small-cell carcinoma is more common than small-cell carcinoma.

NURSING DIAGNOSIS: PAIN

RELATED TO:

- *The presence or growth of the tumor, involvement of lung parenchyma, or surgical incisions*

Nursing Interventions	Rationales
• Assess the patient's level of discomfort, using a pain scale from 0 to 10.	• To help determine measures to take to adequately combat pain
• Monitor vital signs for indications of increased pain, such as rapid heart rate and elevated blood pressure.	• To assess for objective signs of worsening pain
• Address the patient's previous experiences with pain and how the patient coped with them.	• To encourage the use of previously successful coping mechanisms for controlling pain
• Teach the patient nonpharmacologic methods for controlling pain, such as meditation, guided imagery, and therapeutic touch.	• To relieve pain
• Teach the patient about the pharmacologic interventions prescribed for him or her.	• To ensure that the patient knows when to ask for medication to prevent pain from becoming intolerable

NURSING DIAGNOSIS: PAIN *(CONTINUED)*

COLLABORATIVE MANAGEMENT

Interventions	Rationales
• Consult with the pain management specialist about the best modes for treating the patient's pain (for example, when should pain be treated with medication and when should nonpharmacologic pain control methods be used).	• To provide better methods for controlling the pain and discomfort
• Administer medications, as ordered: anti-inflammatories, narcotic analgesics, such as morphine.	• To relieve pain

NURSE ALERT:
Sometimes patients are reluctant to give accurate reports of pain, causing health care providers to underestimate the dosage to prescribe or dispense.

Interventions	Rationales
• Consult with the pain management specialist about the use of patient-controlled analgesia for control of pain.	• To ensure the patient's comfort and to allow the patient active participation in pain management

NURSE ALERT:
Depending on the stage of the patient's illness, pain management may be an important factor in your interventions. Pain medications should be given when needed to ensure patient comfort.

NURSING DIAGNOSIS: PAIN *(CONTINUED)*

OUTCOME:

- The patient will have minimal or no pain.

EVALUATION CRITERIA:

- Pain is reported to be decreased or absent.
- The pain scale rating is 4 or less.

NURSING DIAGNOSES: ANXIETY
FEAR
INEFFECTIVE FAMILY COPING
INEFFECTIVE INDIVIDUAL COPING

RELATED TO:

- *Diagnosis of lung cancer and the eventual outcome of the disease*

Nursing Interventions	Rationales
• Identify the specific areas about which the patient is experiencing fear or anxiety and respond to those concerns.	• To focus interventions on the matters of greatest concern to the patient.
• Answer questions the patient asks about his or her condition, treatment, and related issues, using language appropriate for the patient.	• To alleviate anxiety
• Encourage the patient to use coping skills that have been effective in the past and to develop new ones, if needed.	• To promote the patient's sense of taking an active part in alleviating anxiety
• Supply the patient with information about counseling and support group opportunities.	• To encourage the patient to create a support network to help relieve anxiety
• Assist the patient, family, and caregivers to express their feelings and concerns.	• To help alleviate the patient's anxiety and feelings of isolation

NURSING DIAGNOSES: ANXIETY *(CONTINUED)*

COLLABORATIVE MANAGEMENT

Interventions	Rationales
• Encourage the patient, family, and other caregivers to take advantage of support groups and other social agencies.	• To gain assistance in coping with fear and anxiety

OUTCOME:	EVALUATION CRITERIA:
• The patient will experience manageable levels of anxiety and fear.	• Anxiety and fear are reported to be decreased.
• The patient and family will display healthy coping mechanisms.	• Physical indications of anxiety and fear, such as restlessness, voice tremors, sweating, and elevated respiratory or heart rate are reduced.

NURSING DIAGNOSIS: BODY IMAGE DISTURBANCE

RELATED TO:

- *Altered body structures or function*

Nursing Interventions	Rationales
• Discuss the patient's cancer and feelings about it with him or her. Express your understanding of the feelings and reassure the patient that these feelings are normal.	• To determine the specific areas about which the patient is disturbed
• Allow the patient time to adjust to the condition and allow for temporary expressions of denial or symptoms of withdrawal.	• To allow the patient to develop coping mechanisms

Nursing Interventions *(Continued)*	Rationales *(Continued)*
• Clarify misconceptions about cancer, offer feedback and suggestions, and provide information relevant to the source of the body image disturbance.	• To provide options for the patient to consider and to demonstrate support
• Encourage the patient to take advantage of support groups or other counseling services as appropriate.	• To help the patient develop a support network

COLLABORATIVE MANAGEMENT

Interventions	Rationales
• Consult with the plastic surgery staff about patient's options.	• To provide additional options for the patient
• Discuss the patient's condition with the physical therapy staff to determine if prosthetic devices are appropriate.	• To provide additional options for the patient

OUTCOME:	EVALUATION CRITERIA:
• The patient will be able to accept himself or herself and acquire knowledge about and understanding of the altered body image.	• The patient expresses satisfaction with the choices made for coping with the cancer and its alteration to his or her body.
	• Nonverbal signals indicating body image disturbance, such as social withdrawal, a refusal to look at or touch the body part concerned, or hiding of the body part concerned are absent.

NURSING DIAGNOSIS: KNOWLEDGE DEFICIT

RELATED TO:

- *Unfamiliarity with the disease, treatment plans, self-care routines, and diagnostic tests*

Nursing Interventions	Rationales
• Educate the patient about the pathophysiology of the disease, prescribed medications and their adverse effects, follow-up care requirements, and danger signs that should be reported to the health care provider.	• To increase understanding
• Include the patient's family and other caregivers in the educational program.	• To increase the likelihood that the self-care regimen will be followed
• Encourage the patient to stop smoking, and teach about the effects of secondhand smoke if the patient's family or caregivers are smokers.	• To promote the feeling of control over treatable lung cancer

COLLABORATIVE MANAGEMENT

Interventions	Rationales
• Refer the patient, family, and other caregivers to the appropriate support agencies.	• To encourage understanding of the patient's disease
• Collaborate with other health care providers in stressing the importance of the health care regimen.	• To ensure understanding of the importance of the health care regimen

NURSING DIAGNOSIS: KNOWLEDGE DEFICIT *(CONTINUED)*

OUTCOME:

- The patient will demonstrate adequate knowledge about the disease and self-care routines.

EVALUATION CRITERIA:

- The patient accurately describes the physical effects of the disease.
- The patient verbalizes an understanding of the use of medications, their adverse effects, and danger signs.
- The patient complies with follow-up appointments and the self-care regimen.
- The patient seeks health care if conditions indicate the need.

NURSING DIAGNOSES: IMPAIRED GAS EXCHANGE INEFFECTIVE AIRWAY CLEARANCE INEFFECTIVE BREATHING PATTERN

RELATED TO:

- *Disease progression into terminal stages*

Nursing Interventions	Rationales
• Assess the respiratory pattern for rate, effort, and regularity, and auscultate breath sounds.	• To avoid an increase in respiratory difficulties
• Monitor arterial blood gas values, and assess for other signs of impaired gas exchange, such as decreasing arterial pulse oximetry, changes in level of consciousness, and restlessness.	• To prevent inadequate gas exchange
• Instruct the patient in effective breathing patterns, and assist him or her to maintain a comfortable position, such as sitting up in the orthopneic position.	• To ease respiratory efforts

NURSING DIAGNOSES: IMPAIRED GAS EXCHANGE *(CONTINUED)*

Nursing Interventions *(Continued)*	Rationales *(Continued)*
• Encourage the patient to clear secretions from the lungs, if possible.	• To promote adequate respiration
• Use room humidifiers to increase the patient's ability to clear lung secretions by keeping the secretions moist.	• To promote adequate respiration and clearance of secretions

COLLABORATIVE MANAGEMENT

Interventions	Rationales
• Consult with the respiratory therapy staff if indicated by the patient's condition.	• To develop an effective care plan for dealing with the patient's respiration problems

OUTCOME:

- The patient will maintain easy, relaxed breathing and effective ventilation.

EVALUATION CRITERIA:

- Breathing pattern is regular and easy.
- There are no signs of respiratory distress.
- Arterial blood gas values are within normal ranges.
- There is no evidence of cyanosis.

NURSING DIAGNOSIS: ALTERED NUTRITION (LESS THAN BODY REQUIREMENTS)

RELATED TO:

- *Therapeutic regimen or metastasis of the tumor*

Nursing Interventions	Rationales
• Obtain admission weight and monitor weight on a weekly basis.	• To use in monitoring the therapeutic regimen

Nursing Interventions *(Continued)*	Rationales *(Continued)*
• Inquire about the patient's favorite foods and eating habits, and encourage patient involvement in food choices and nutritional management.	• To develop a useful diet plan for use during and after therapy
• Promote a favorable atmosphere for eating, and eliminate barriers to pleasurable eating, such as unpleasant odors or tastes and scheduling meals when the patient is tired.	• To reduce resistance to eating and encourage adequate nutritional intake
• Encourage the patient to eat frequent, small meals.	• To avoid fatigue and a feeling of overfullness
• Encourage the patient to consume high-calorie, high-protein snacks and to take supplements.	• To get maximum protein and calories with a minimum expenditure of effort

COLLABORATIVE MANAGEMENT

Interventions	Rationales
• Consult with the dietitian to obtain an accurate assessment of the patient's nutritional requirements.	• To aid in developing an appropriate diet plan

OUTCOME:	EVALUATION CRITERIA:
• The patient will have adequate nutritional intake to maintain body weight at or around admission weight.	• Laboratory test results, such as pre-albumen levels and transferrin levels, indicate proper nutritional support. • Weight is within the range of admission weight.

NURSING DIAGNOSIS: HIGH RISK FOR INFECTION

RELATED TO:

- *Surgical procedures for diagnosis or treatment of the disease and decreased immunity related to the stress of the illness*

Nursing Interventions	Rationales
• Monitor vital signs for changes that indicate infection, such as elevated temperature and rapid heart rate.	• To prevent onset or worsening of infection
• Encourage the patient to drink fluids, maintain adequate nutrition, and rest frequently.	• To prevent onset or worsening of infection
• Teach the patient basic infection control practices, such as hand washing and avoidance of other infected people.	• To minimize the risk of contracting infection

COLLABORATIVE MANAGEMENT

Interventions	Rationales
• Administer medications, as ordered: antibiotics.	• To reduce or eliminate infection

NURSE ALERT:
Be careful to assess the patient for adverse reactions to drugs and food.

Interventions	Rationales
• Maintain good infection control procedures for staff and visitors, including reverse isolation, if needed, the use of gowns and masks, and other requirements as established by your facility.	• To reduce the risk of infection

NURSING DIAGNOSIS: HIGH RISK FOR INFECTION *(CONTINUED)*

OUTCOME:

- The patient will be free of signs of infection.

EVALUATION CRITERIA:

- Vital signs are normal.
- Indications of infection at the incision site, such as redness, swelling, or purulent drainage are absent.

NURSING DIAGNOSIS: ALTERED TISSUE INTEGRITY

RELATED TO:

- *Treatment for malignant conditions*

Nursing Interventions	Rationales
• Assess the patient's skin for color, turgor, temperature, and texture.	• To determine appropriate interventions
• Moisturize the patient's skin with nonirritating lotions or creams.	• To prevent infection and damage to the skin and reduce tissue sloughing
• Avoid the use of extreme heat or cold, such as hot water for cleaning or ice packs or heating pads.	• To avoid undue irritation of the skin
• Instruct the patient to limit exposure to the sun and to use adequate protection (at least SPF 15).	• To avoid damage from sunburn and to reduce sensitivity that may be caused by treatments

COLLABORATIVE MANAGEMENT

Interventions	Rationales
• Administer medications as ordered: analgesics, antibiotic ointments.	• To ease discomfort caused by skin irritation and to reduce the risk of infection

NURSING DIAGNOSIS: ALTERED TISSUE INTEGRITY *(CONTINUED)*

OUTCOME:	EVALUATION CRITERIA:
• The patient's skin will be warm, dry, and intact.	• The patient's skin is normal in color, turgor, and temperature. • There are no signs of edema or erythema.

NURSING DIAGNOSIS: NONCOMPLIANCE

RELATED TO:

- *Denial of the condition, difficulties involved in lifestyle changes required to accommodate the condition, and lack of knowledge about the disease and required changes*

Nursing Interventions	Rationales
• Determine the nature of the patient's noncompliance through discussion with the patient and his or her family or other caregivers, if possible and appropriate.	• To determine areas on which to focus your interventions
• Listen to the patient's reasons for noncompliance. Respond in a nonjudgmental manner.	• To encourage the patient to express his or her concerns and to emphasize that you respect the patient's opinions and right to make decisions about care and treatment
• Provide appropriate information about lifestyle changes, treatment options, the patient's condition, and coping techniques.	• To increase patient knowledge
• Develop a contract with the patient to identify tasks the patient will do, changes he or she will make (such as smoking cessation and weight management), and goals the patient will attempt to meet.	• To increase patient participation in acceptable activities, thereby increasing overall compliance

COLLABORATIVE MANAGEMENT

Interventions	Rationales
• Explain the patient's decisions to other staff members. Document the patient's decisions carefully.	• To identify the ways in which other staff members may have to alter their care plans and activities
• Collaborate with other health care providers in stressing the importance of the health care regimen.	• To ensure understanding of the importance of the health care regimen
• Encourage the patient to participate in discussions with other patients who are coping with the same problems, limitations, and challenges.	• To provide an opportunity for the patient to learn new methods for coping with bronchitis or emphysema and thereby increase the potential for patient compliance

NURSE ALERT:
Remember that it is the patient's right to refuse treatment or to participate in a care plan and you must respect that right, provided it does not endanger you, other staff members, or other patients.

OUTCOME:	EVALUATION CRITERIA:
• The patient will complete self-care activities and participate in treatment, as established by mutual agreement.	• The patient enters into a care and treatment contract. • The patient complies with follow-up appointments and self-care regimen, as defined.

Patient Teaching

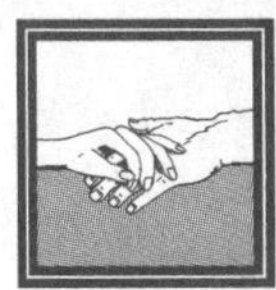

Although the prognosis for patients with lung cancer is usually poor, education should center around quality-of-life issues and care should center around meeting the patient's needs for comfort, counseling, and adapting to the changes made necessary by the disease.

Inform the patient about the choices he or she can make to ease symptoms: smoking cessation, nutritional support, and therapy options.

When necessary, encourage the patient to make use of support groups and individual and family counseling to ease anxiety and fear and enhance coping skills.

Documentation

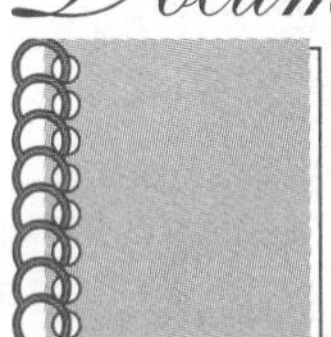

- Admission weight
- Laboratory test results
- Patient compliance with care regimen

Nursing Research

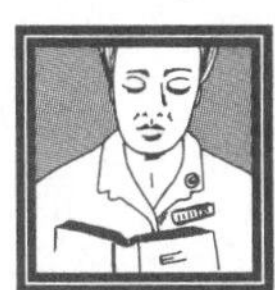

Effective care of the patient with lung cancer must include not only medical attention to the patient's physical needs but also a wide variety of issues such as employment and finances, the psychosocial needs of the patient as well as those of the family and other caregivers, and the adaptations the patient must make to a life in the shadow of cancer.

Seale, D. D., and B. M. Beaver. "Pathophysiology of Lung Cancer." *Nursing Clinics of North America* 27 (September 1992): 603–613.

Chapter 13. Cancers of the Head and Neck

▽ ▽ ▽ ▽ ▽ ▽ ▽

Introduction

Cancers of the head and neck are primarily the result of the lifestyle and health habit choices a person makes. Contributing factors include exposure to tobacco and smoke as well as to alcohol. These conditions include cancer of the oral cavity, oropharynx, larynx, hypopharynx, esophagus, nasal cavity, sinuses, nasopharynx, and salivary glands.

NURSING DIAGNOSIS: PAIN

RELATED TO:

- *Presence or growth of the tumor or to surgical incisions*

Nursing Interventions	Rationales
• Assess the patient's level of discomfort, using a pain scale from 0 to 10.	• To help determine measures to take to adequately combat pain
• Monitor vital signs for indications of increased pain, such as rapid heart rate and elevated blood pressure.	• To assess for objective signs of worsening pain
• Address the patient's previous experiences with pain and how the patient coped with them.	• To encourage the use of previously successful coping mechanisms for controlling pain
• Teach the patient nonpharmacologic methods for controlling pain, such as meditation, guided imagery, and therapeutic touch.	• To relieve pain
• Teach the patient about the pharmacologic interventions prescribed for him or her.	• To ensure that the patient knows when to ask for medication to prevent pain from becoming intolerable

NURSING DIAGNOSIS: PAIN *(CONTINUED)*

COLLABORATIVE MANAGEMENT

Interventions	Rationales
• Consult the pain management specialist about the best modes for treating the patient's pain (for example, when should pain be treated with medication or when should nonpharmacologic pain control methods be used).	• To provide better methods for controlling pain and discomfort
• Administer medications, as ordered: anti-inflammatories, narcotic analgesics (such as morphine).	• To relieve pain

NURSE ALERT:
Sometimes patients are reluctant to give accurate reports of pain, causing health care providers to underestimate the dosage to prescribe or dispense.

Interventions	Rationales
• Consult the pain management specialist about the use of patient-controlled analgesia for control of pain.	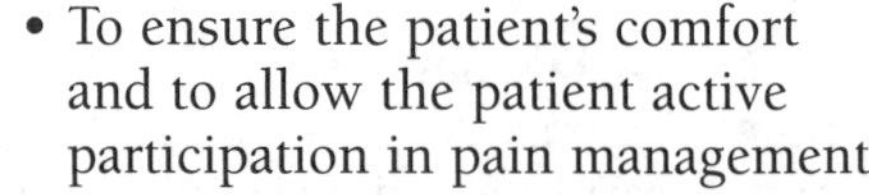 • To ensure the patient's comfort and to allow the patient active participation in pain management

NURSE ALERT:
Depending on the stage of the patient's illness, pain management may be an important factor in your interventions. Pain medications should be given when needed to ensure patient comfort. Some patients may require round-the-clock medication to control pain.

NURSING DIAGNOSIS: PAIN *(CONTINUED)*

OUTCOME:	EVALUATION CRITERIA:
• The patient will have minimal or no pain.	• Pain is reported to be decreased or absent.
	• The pain scale rating is 4 or less.

NURSING DIAGNOSES: ANXIETY
FEAR
INEFFECTIVE FAMILY COPING
INEFFECTIVE INDIVIDUAL COPING

RELATED TO:

• *Diagnosis of cancer and the eventual outcome of the disease*

Nursing Interventions	Rationales
• Identify the specific areas about which the patient is experiencing fear or anxiety and respond to those concerns.	• To focus interventions on the matters of greatest concern to the patient
• Answer questions the patient asks about his or her cancer, treatment, and related issues, using language appropriate for the patient.	• To alleviate anxiety
• Encourage the patient to use coping skills that have been effective in the past and to develop new ones, if needed.	• To promote the sense of taking an active part in alleviating anxiety
• Supply the patient with information about counseling and support group opportunities.	• To encourage the patient to create a support network to help relieve anxiety
• Assist the patient, family, and caregivers to express their feelings and concerns.	• To alleviate anxiety

NURSING DIAGNOSES: ANXIETY *(CONTINUED)*

COLLABORATIVE MANAGEMENT

Interventions	Rationales
• Encourage the patient, family, and other caregivers to take advantage of support groups and other social agencies.	• To gain assistance in coping with fear and anxiety

OUTCOME:	EVALUATION CRITERIA:
• The patient will experience manageable levels of anxiety and fear.	• Anxiety and fear are reported to be decreased.
• The patient and family will display healthy coping mechanisms.	• Physical indications of anxiety and fear, such as restlessness, voice tremors, sweating, and elevated respiratory or heart rate are reduced.

NURSING DIAGNOSIS: BODY IMAGE DISTURBANCE

RELATED TO:

• *Altered body structures or function*

Nursing Intervention	Rationale
• Discuss the patient's cancer and feelings about it with him or her. Express your understanding of the feelings and reassure the patient that these feelings are normal.	• To determine the specific areas about which the patient is disturbed
• Allow the patient time to adjust to the condition and allow for temporary expressions of denial or symptoms of withdrawal.	• To allow patient to develop coping mechanisms

Nursing Intervention *(Continued)*	Rationales *(Continued)*
• Clarify misconceptions about cancer, offer feedback and suggestions, and provide information relevant to the source of the body image disturbance.	• To provide options for the patient to consider and to demonstrate support
• Encourage the patient to take advantage of support groups or other counseling services as appropriate.	• To help the patient develop a support network

COLLABORATIVE MANAGEMENT

Interventions	Rationales
• Consult with plastic surgery staff about patient's options.	• To provide additional options for the patient
• Discuss patient's condition with physical therapy staff to determine if prosthetic devices are appropriate.	• To provide additional options for the patient

OUTCOME:	EVALUATION CRITERIA:
• The patient will be able to accept himself or herself and acquire knowledge about and understanding of the altered body image.	• The patient expresses satisfaction with the choices made for coping with the cancer and its alteration to his or her body. • Nonverbal signals indicating body image disturbance, such as social withdrawal, a refusal to look at or touch the body part concerned, or hiding of the body part concerned are absent.

NURSING DIAGNOSIS: KNOWLEDGE DEFICIT

RELATED TO:

- *Unfamiliarity with the disease, treatment plans, self-care routines, and diagnostic tests*

Nursing Interventions	Rationales
• Educate the patient about the pathophysiology of the disease, prescribed medications and their adverse effects, follow-up care requirements, and danger signs that should be reported to the health care provider.	• To increase understanding
• Include the patient's family and other caregivers in the educational program.	• To increase the likelihood that the self-care regimen will be followed
• Encourage the patient to stop smoking, and teach the patient about the effects of secondhand smoke if the patient's family and caregivers are smokers.	• To encourage the feeling of control over treatable lung cancer

COLLABORATIVE MANAGEMENT

Interventions	Rationales
• Refer the patient, family, and other caregivers to the appropriate support agencies.	• To encourage understanding of the patient's condition
• Collaborate with other health care providers in stressing the importance of the health care regimen.	• To ensure understanding of the importance of the health care regimen

OUTCOME:	EVALUATION CRITERIA:
• The patient will demonstrate adequate knowledge about the disease and self-care routines.	• The patient accurately describes the physical effects of the disease.

NURSING DIAGNOSIS: KNOWLEDGE DEFICIT *(CONTINUED)*

OUTCOME:
(Continued)

- The patient will demonstrate adequate knowledge about the disease and self-care routines. *(continued)*

EVALUATION CRITERIA:
(Continued)

- The patient verbalizes an understanding of the use of medications, their adverse effects, and danger signs.
- The patient complies with follow-up appointments and the self-care regimen.
- The patient seeks health care if conditions indicate the need.

NURSING DIAGNOSES: IMPAIRED GAS EXCHANGE INEFFECTIVE AIRWAY CLEARANCE INEFFECTIVE BREATHING PATTERN

RELATED TO:

- *Disease progression into terminal stages*

Nursing Interventions	Rationales
• Assess respiratory patterns for rate, effort, and regularity, and auscultate breath sounds.	• To prevent an increase in respiratory difficulties
• Monitor arterial blood gas values, and assess for other signs of inefficient gas exchange.	• To prevent inadequate gas exchange
• Instruct the patient in effective breathing pattern, and assist him or her to maintain a comfortable position.	• To ease respiratory efforts
• Encourage the patient to clear secretions from the lungs, if possible.	• To promote adequate respiration
• Use room humidifiers to increase the patient's ability to clear lung secretions by keeping the secretions moist.	• To promote adequate respiration and clearance of secretions

NURSING DIAGNOSES: IMPAIRED GAS EXCHANGE *(CONTINUED)*

COLLABORATIVE MANAGEMENT

Interventions	Rationales
• Consult with the respiratory therapy staff if indicated by the patient's condition.	• To develop an effective care plan for dealing with the patient's respiration problems

OUTCOME:	EVALUATION CRITERIA:
• The patient will maintain easy, relaxed breathing and effective ventilation.	• Breathing patterns are regular and easy. • There are no signs of respiratory distress. • Arterial blood gas values are normal. • There is no evidence of cyanosis.

NURSING DIAGNOSIS: ALTERED NUTRITION (LESS THAN BODY REQUIREMENTS)

RELATED TO:

• *Therapeutic regimen or metastasis of the tumor*

Nursing Interventions	Rationales
• Obtain admission weight and monitor weight on a weekly basis.	• To use in monitoring the therapeutic regimen
• Inquire about the patient's favorite foods and eating habits, and encourage patient involvement in food choices and nutritional management.	• To develop a useful diet plan for use during and after therapy

Nursing Interventions *(Continued)*	Rationales *(Continued)*
• Promote a favorable atmosphere for eating and eliminate barriers to pleasurable eating, such as unpleasant odors or tastes and scheduling meals when the patient is tired.	• To reduce resistance to eating and encourage adequate nutritional intake
• Encourage the patient to eat frequent, small meals.	• To avoid fatigue and a feeling of overfullness
• Encourage the patient to consume high-calorie, high-protein snacks and to take supplements.	• To get maximum protein and calories with a minimum expenditure of effort

COLLABORATIVE MANAGEMENT

Interventions	Rationales
• Consult with the dietitian for an accurate assessment of the patient's nutritional requirements.	• To aid in developing an appropriate diet plan

OUTCOME:	EVALUATION CRITERIA:
• The patient will have adequate nutritional intake to maintain body weight at or around admission weight.	• Laboratory test results, such as pre-albumen levels and transferrin levels, indicate proper nutritional support. • Weight is within the range of admission weight.

NURSING DIAGNOSIS: HIGH RISK FOR INFECTION

RELATED TO:

- *Surgical procedures for the diagnosis or treatment of the disease and decreased immunity related to the stress of the illness*

Nursing Interventions	Rationales
• Monitor vital signs for changes that indicate infection, such as elevated temperature and rapid heart rate.	• To prevent onset or worsening of infection

NURSING DIAGNOSIS: HIGH RISK FOR INFECTION *(CONTINUED)*

Nursing Interventions (Continued)	Rationales *(Continued)*
• Encourage the patient to drink fluids (1,500 to 2,000 mL daily), maintain adequate nutrition, and rest frequently.	• To prevent onset or worsening of infection
• Teach the patient basic infection control practices, such as hand washing and avoidance of other infected people.	• To minimize the risk of contracting infection

COLLABORATIVE MANAGEMENT

Interventions	Rationales
• Administer medications, as ordered: antibiotics.	• To reduce or eliminate infection

NURSE ALERT:
Be careful to assess the patient for adverse reactions to drugs and food.

Interventions	Rationales
• Prepare the patient, if necessary, for surgery.	• To control infection

OUTCOME:
- The patient will be free of signs of infection.

EVALUATION CRITERIA:
- Vital signs are normal.
- Indications of infection at the incision site, such as redness, swelling, or purulent drainage, are absent.

NURSING DIAGNOSIS: ALTERED TISSUE INTEGRITY

RELATED TO:

- *Treatment for malignant conditions*

Nursing Interventions	Rationales
• Assess the patient's skin for color, turgor, temperature, and texture.	• To determine appropriate interventions
• Moisturize the patient's skin with nonirritating lotions or creams.	• To prevent infection and damage to the skin and reduce tissue sloughing
• Avoid the use of extreme heat or cold, such as hot water for cleaning or ice packs or heating pads.	• To avoid undue irritation of the skin
• Instruct the patient to limit exposure to the sun and to use adequate protection (at least SPF 15).	• To avoid damage from sunburn and to reduce sensitivity that may be caused by treatments

COLLABORATIVE MANAGEMENT

Interventions	Rationales
• Administer medications as ordered: analgesics, antibiotic ointments.	• To ease discomfort caused by skin irritation and to reduce the risk of infection

OUTCOME:	EVALUATION CRITERIA:
• The patient's skin will be warm, dry, and intact.	• The patient's skin is normal in color, turgor, and temperature.
	• There are no signs of edema or erythema.

NURSING DIAGNOSIS: NONCOMPLIANCE

RELATED TO:

- *Denial of the condition, difficulties involved in lifestyle changes required to accommodate the condition, and lack of knowledge about the disease and required changes*

Nursing Interventions	Rationales
• Determine the nature of the patient's noncompliance through discussion with the patient and his or her family or other caregivers, if possible and appropriate.	• To determine areas on which to focus your interventions
• Listen to the patient's reasons for noncompliance. Respond in a nonjudgmental manner.	• To encourage the patient to express his or her concerns and to emphasize that you respect the patient's opinions and right to make decisions about care and treatment
• Provide appropriate information about lifestyle changes, treatment options, the patient's condition, and coping techniques.	• To increase the patient's knowledge
• Develop a contract with the patient to identify tasks the patient will do, changes he or she will make (such as smoking cessation and weight management), and goals the patient will attempt to meet.	• To increase patient participation in acceptable activities, thereby increasing overall compliance

NURSE ALERT:
Remember that it is the patient's right to refuse treatment or to participate in a care plan and you must respect that right, provided it does not endanger you, other staff members, or other patients.

COLLABORATIVE MANAGEMENT

Interventions	Rationales
• Explain the patient's decisions to other staff members. Document the patient's decisions carefully.	• To identify the ways in which other staff members may have to alter their care plans and activities
• Collaborate with other health care providers in stressing the importance of the health care regimen.	• To ensure understanding of the importance of the health care regimen
• Encourage the patient to participate in discussions with other patients who are coping with the same problems, limitations, and challenges.	• To provide an opportunity for the patient to learn new methods for coping with bronchitis or emphysema and thereby increase the potential for patient compliance

OUTCOME:	EVALUATION CRITERIA:
• The patient will complete self-care activities and participate in treatment, as established by mutual agreement.	• The patient enters into a care and treatment contract. • The patient complies with follow-up appointments and self-care regimen, as defined.

Patient Teaching

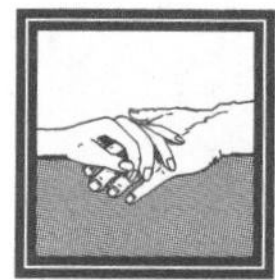

Patient teaching should center around the lifestyle changes a person can make to reduce the risk of cancer of the head and neck.

Additional teaching should address the issues of patient appearance, if the disease or treatment causes disfigurement.

When necessary, encourage the patient to make use of group, individual, and family counseling to ease fear and enhance coping skills.

Documentation

- Admission weight
- Laboratory test results
- Patient compliance with care regimen

Suggested Readings

Houston, S. J., and J. A. Kendall. "Psychosocial Implications of Lung Cancer." *Nursing Clinics of North America* 27, no. 3 (1992): 681–690.

Lockhart, J. S., J. L. Troff, and L. S. Arton. "A Case Study: Total Laryngectomy and Radical Neck Dissection." *American Operating Room Nurse Journal* 55, no. 2 (1992): 458–479.

McQuirrie, D. G. "Head and Neck Cancer—An Overview for the Perioperative Nurse." *American Operating Room Nurse Journal* 56, no. 7 (1992): 79–97.

Schmitt, R. "Quality of Life Issues in Lung Cancer: New Symptom Management Strategies." *Chest* 103, no. 1 (1993): 515–545.

SECTION VI. RESPIRATORY EMERGENCIES

Chapter 14. Pneumothorax and Hemothorax

▽ ▽ ▽ ▽ ▽ ▽ ▽

Introduction

SEE TEXT PAGES ________

Pneumothorax is the accumulation of air in the pleural space and is frequently associated with chest trauma. Spontaneous pneumothorax may be related to chronic obstructive pulmonary disease or other pulmonary disease. Iatrogenic pneumothorax may be created by several diagnostic and therapeutic procedures. Hemothorax is the accumulation of blood in the pleural space.

DIAGRAM OF INTACT LUNG PLEURA

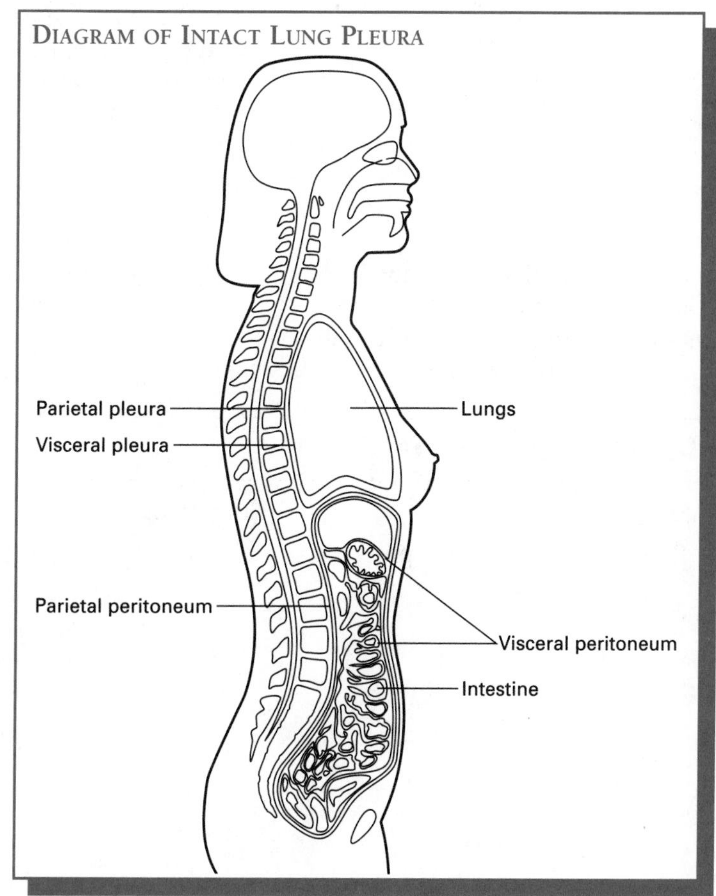

NURSING DIAGNOSES: IMPAIRED GAS EXCHANGE INEFFECTIVE BREATHING PATTERN

RELATED TO:

- *Respiratory emergency and the compromised integrity of pulmonary structures*

Nursing Interventions	Rationales
• Observe the patient's chest expansion, tracheal alignment, vital signs, respiratory status (rate effort and regularity), arterial blood gas values, pulse oximetry, and chest radiographs closely.	• To detect evidence of pneumothorax or development of tension pneumothorax  **NURSE ALERT:** Tension pneumothorax is indicated by decreased chest expansion on the affected side, tracheal deviation away from the affected side, decreased blood pressure, and rapid heart rate. Immediate intervention, in the form of thoracentesis or chest tube placement, is required.
• Assist the patient to maintain a comfortable position for maximum respiratory benefit, usually high Fowler's position.	• To ease respiration and facilitate diaphragmatic excursion.

COLLABORATIVE MANAGEMENT

Interventions	Rationales
• Prepare the patient for phlebotomy, if indicated.	• To decrease venous pressure
• Administer oxygen therapy, as ordered.	• To decrease tissue hypoxia
• Monitor arterial blood gas values and pulse oximetry.	• To detect signs of respiratory failure

COLLABORATIVE MANAGEMENT *(CONTINUED)*

Interventions *(Continued)*	Rationales *(Continued)*
• Administer medications as ordered: analgesics, sedatives.	• To aid respiratory effort
• Prepare the patient for diagnostic or therapeutic measures, such as chest tube insertion and thoracentesis for pneumothorax or tension pneumothorax and lung perfusion and ventilation scans and pulmonary angiography for pulmonary embolism.	• To ensure ventilation and protect the airway
• If the patient is intubated, suction the airway as needed. Use sterile saline instillations to clear the secretions, if required.	• To ensure adequate respiration and ease the clearing of secretions

OUTCOME:	EVALUATION CRITERIA:
• The patient will be able to sustain spontaneous ventilation with an easy, regular pattern. Adequate ventilation will occur.	• Breathing is relaxed and easy. • Vital signs are within normal limits. • Arterial blood gas values are normal. • There is no evidence of cyanosis.

NURSING DIAGNOSES: ANXIETY
FEAR

RELATED TO:

- *Uncertain outcome of the disorder, dyspnea and other respiratory difficulties, pain, and lack of information about the disorder, treatment plans, diagnostics tests, and procedures*

Nursing Interventions	Rationales
• Explain the disorder to the patient and family members or other caregivers, using appropriate language.	• To ease unfamiliarity and discomfort

NURSING DIAGNOSES: ANXIETY *(CONTINUED)*

Nursing Interventions *(Continued)*	Rationales *(Continued)*
• Monitor the patient for signs of increasing distress.	• To prevent levels of anxiety and fear from becoming an additional burden on the patient's condition
• Maintain a calm, relaxed demeanor, and reassure the patient that his or her condition is monitored at all times.	• To prevent additional anxiety concerning the staff's presence and attitude
• Encourage the patient to share his or her concerns, and respond to each as appropriate.	• To maintain open lines of communication
• Promote a quiet environment by reducing external stimulation.	• To limit the drain on the patient's resources—mental, emotional, and physical
• Plan for care activities at times when the patient is feeling best able to handle the stress.	• To avoid unduly stressing the patient

COLLABORATIVE MANAGEMENT

Interventions	Rationales
• Administer medications as ordered: analgesics, antianxiety agents, sedatives.	• To decrease the patient's anxiety and fear and relieve pain or discomfort
• Encourage the patient and family to take advantage of counseling services and support groups, as appropriate.	• To develop effective coping skills

OUTCOME:	EVALUATION CRITERIA:
• The patient will appear calm and relaxed.	• Physical signs of distress, such as agitation, restlessness, and elevated respiratory rate are decreased or absent. • Confidence and relaxation are increased.

NURSING DIAGNOSIS: KNOWLEDGE DEFICIT

RELATED TO:

- *Patient's disorder, treatment plans, diagnostic tests, and procedures*

Nursing Interventions	Rationales
• Explain, using appropriate language, the patient's disorder.	• To increase awareness of the patient's disorder
• Encourage the patient, family members, and other caregivers to ask questions.	• To reinforce their understanding of the patient's disorder and treatment procedures
• Teach the patient necessary self-care routines, as required.	• To promote the feeling of control over the situation
• Explain prescribed medications and their adverse effects, including danger signs that the patient should report to the health care provider.	• To increase understanding of the therapeutic measures
• Describe the danger signs and symptoms that the patient should report to the health care provider, such as difficulty in breathing, especially when lying down or with exertion.	• To increase understanding of the patient's disorder and prevent a respiratory emergency

COLLABORATIVE MANAGEMENT

Interventions	Rationales
• Confer with physicians and other health care providers to identify other situations the patient may experience in the course of treatment.	• To anticipate the patient's need for information and to provide for it before the patient finds himself or herself in an anxiety-producing situation

OUTCOME:	EVALUATION CRITERIA:
• The patient will demonstrate increased understanding of his or her disorder.	• The patient describes the disorder, treatment plans, prescribed medications and adverse effects, and danger signs and symptoms.

NURSING DIAGNOSIS: PAIN

RELATED TO:

- *Injury or trauma, iatrogenic devices needed to ensure respiration and ventilation, or surgical procedures required by the patient's disorder*

Nursing Interventions	Rationales
• Assess the patient's level of discomfort, using a pain scale from 0 to 10.	• To help determine measures to take to adequately combat pain
• Monitor vital signs for indications of increased pain, such as rapid heart rate and elevated blood pressure.	• To assess for objective signs of worsening pain
• Address the patient's previous experiences with pain and how the patient coped with them.	• To encourage the use of previously successful coping mechanisms for controlling pain
• Teach the patient nonpharmacologic methods for controlling pain, such as meditation, guided imagery, and therapeutic touch.	• To relieve pain
• Teach patient about the pharmacologic interventions prescribed for him or her.	• To ensure that the patient knows when to ask for medication to prevent pain from becoming intolerable

COLLABORATIVE MANAGEMENT

Interventions	Rationales
• Consult with the pain management specialist about the best modes for treating the patient's pain (for example, when should pain be treated with medication and when should nonpharmacologic pain control methods be used).	• To provide better methods for controlling the pain and discomfort

COLLABORATIVE MANAGEMENT *(CONTINUED)*

Interventions *(Continued)*	Rationales *(Continued)*
• Administer medications, as ordered: analgesics.	• To relieve pain

NURSE ALERT:
Sometimes patients are reluctant to give accurate reports of pain, causing health care providers to underestimate the dosage to prescribe or dispense.

OUTCOME:	EVALUATION CRITERIA:
• The patient will have minimal or no pain.	• Pain or discomfort is reported to be decreased or absent. • The pain scale rating is 4 or less.

NURSING DIAGNOSIS: HIGH RISK FOR INFECTION

RELATED TO:
- *Trauma or injury or to iatrogenic devices needed to ensure adequate lung expansion*

Nursing Interventions	Rationales
• Monitor the patient for signs of increasing infection, including evaluation of sputum, if appropriate.	• To prevent infection from occurring or worsening
• Monitor the chest tube insertion site for redness, swelling, and tenderness.	• To prevent infection from occurring or worsening
• Monitor chest tube drainage for amount, color, and character.	• To identify the need to increase or initiate suction

NURSING DIAGNOSIS: HIGH RISK FOR INFECTION *(CONTINUED)*

Nursing Interventions *(Continued)*	Rationales *(Continued)*
• If the patient is intubated, institute an appropriate hygiene regimen and good pulmonary toilet, including chest physiotherapy and aseptic suctioning techniques.	• To decrease the likelihood of infection
• Encourage the patient to clear secretions from the respiratory passageways and, if needed, suction the secretions. If the patient is not intubated, use deep breathing, cough, and incentive spirometry.	• To reduce the accumulation of secretions, which can lead to infection

COLLABORATIVE MANAGEMENT

Interventions	Rationales
• Administer medications, as ordered: antibiotics.	• To reduce and resolve infection
• Submit drainage samples for microscopic evaluation.	• To detect signs of infection

OUTCOME:	EVALUATION CRITERIA:
• The patient will remain free of infection, and the chest tube insertion site, if present, will show no signs of infection.	• Vital signs and white blood cell count are normal. Pleural fluid cultures are negative. • Surgical incision or injury, if present, shows no signs of swelling or redness.

NURSING DIAGNOSIS: DECREASED CARDIAC OUTPUT

RELATED TO:

- *Unresolved tension pneumothorax*

Nursing Interventions	Rationales
• Monitor the patient for signs of cardiac distress, including decreasing mental status, decreasing blood pressure, increasing heart rate and rhythm, unequal chest expansion, and tracheal deviation.	• To anticipate the need for resuscitative measures
• Assure that emergency resuscitative equipment is readily available for immediate use.	• To promote fast, effective treatment
• Prepare the patient for therapeutic measures, such as chest tube insertion and thoracentesis for pneumothorax or tension pneumothorax.	• To relieve pressure on the heart and great vessels and help restore cardiac output

COLLABORATIVE MANAGEMENT

Interventions	Rationales
• Assist with diagnostic procedures, especially pulmonary artery catheterization and central venous pressure monitoring.	• To provide accurate information for use by the staff, if needed
• Initiate oxygen therapy, as ordered.	• To prevent tissue hypoxia
• Monitor arterial blood gas values and pulse oximetry.	• To identify signs of respiratory failure

NURSING DIAGNOSIS: DECREASED CARDIAC OUTPUT

(CONTINUED)

OUTCOME:

- The patient will maintain adequate cardiac output for his or her age and body surface area.

EVALUATION CRITERIA:

- Blood pressure is normal.
- Pulse rate is strong and regular.
- Mental status is clear.
- Heartbeat pattern is normal.
- Jugular vein is not distended.

Patient Teaching

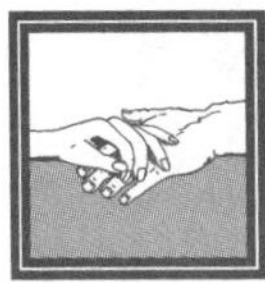

Patient teaching in respiratory emergency situations initially centers around the patient's condition and prognosis. Teaching may be directed toward the patient, if his or her condition permits, or toward the patient's family or other caregivers.

Explain that in most cases, once the patient has been stabilized, the lungs will re-expand within 48 to 72 hours.

Educate the patient and family about treatment plans, monitoring, and diagnostic procedures and tests.

When the patient is ready for discharge, instruct the patient in self-care routines, activity restrictions, and the proper use of prescribed medications. Reinforce information about danger signs that should be reported to the health care provider and any special dietary or activity restrictions.

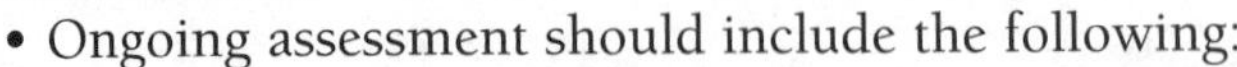

Documentation

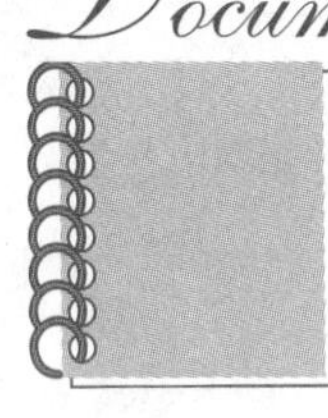

- Ongoing assessment should include the following:
  - Vital signs, especially respiratory rate, effort, and pattern
  - Arterial blood gas analysis
  - Radiography
  - Pulse oximetry
  - Daily weight
- Patient compliance with care regimen
- Patient response to prescribed medications and other therapeutic measures

Chapter 15. Chest Injuries

Introduction

SEE TEXT PAGES ______

Chest injuries are grouped into two main categories: penetrating and nonpenetrating, or blunt, injury. In both cases, complications such as hemothorax, pneumothorax, shock, diaphragmatic rupture, and pulmonary contusion are common.

NURSING DIAGNOSES: IMPAIRED GAS EXCHANGE INEFFECTIVE BREATHING PATTERN

RELATED TO:

- *Respiratory emergency and the compromised integrity of pulmonary structures*

Nursing Interventions	Rationales
• Observe the patient's chest expansion, tracheal alignment, vital signs, respiratory status (rate effort and regularity), arterial blood gas values, pulse oximetry, and chest radiographs closely. Auscultate breath sounds frequently (every 15 minutes).	• To determine current level of respiratory function  **NURSE ALERT:** Tension pneumothorax is indicated by decreased chest expansion on the affected side, tracheal deviation away from the affected side, decreased blood pressure, and rapid heart rate. Immediate intervention, in the form of thoracentesis or chest tube placement, is required.
• Assist the patient to maintain a comfortable position for maximum respiratory benefit, usually high Fowler's position.	• To ease respiration and facilitate diaphragmatic excursion

NURSING DIAGNOSES: IMPAIRED GAS EXCHANGE *(CONTINUED)*

COLLABORATIVE MANAGEMENT

Interventions	Rationales
• Administer oxygen therapy, as ordered.	• To decrease tissue hypoxia
• Monitor arterial blood gas values and pulse oximetry.	• To detect signs of respiratory failure
• Administer medications as ordered: analgesics, bronchodilators, sedatives.	• To aid respiratory effort and to decrease pain
• Prepare the patient for diagnostic or therapeutic measures, such as chest tube insertion and thoracentesis for pneumothorax or tension pneumothorax and lung perfusion and ventilation scans, if indicated.	• To ensure ventilation and protect the airway
• If the patient is intubated, suction the airway as needed. Use sterile saline instillations to clear the secretions, if required.	• To ensure adequate respiration and ease the clearing of secretions

OUTCOME:

- The patient will be able to sustain spontaneous ventilation with an easy, regular pattern. Adequate ventilation will occur.

EVALUATION CRITERIA:

- Breathing is relaxed and easy.
- Vital signs are within normal limits.
- Arterial blood gas values are normal.
- There is no evidence of cyanosis.

NURSING DIAGNOSES: ANXIETY FEAR

RELATED TO:

- *Uncertain outcome of the disorder, dyspnea and other respiratory difficulties, pain, and lack of information about the disorder, treatment plans, diagnostics tests, and procedures*

Nursing Interventions	Rationales
• Explain the disorder to the patient and family members or other caregivers, using appropriate language.	• To ease unfamiliarity and discomfort
• Monitor the patient for signs of increasing distress.	• To prevent levels of anxiety and fear from becoming an additional burden on the patient's condition
• Maintain a calm, relaxed demeanor, and reassure the patient that his or her condition is monitored at all times.	• To prevent additional anxiety concerning the staff's presence and attitude
• Encourage the patient to share his or her concerns, and respond to each as appropriate.	• To maintain open lines of communication
• Promote a quiet environment by reducing external stimulation.	• To limit the drain on the patient's resources—mental, emotional, and physical
• Plan for care activities at times when the patient is feeling best able to handle the stress.	• To avoid unduly stressing the patient

COLLABORATIVE MANAGEMENT

Interventions	Rationales
• Administer medications as ordered: analgesics, antianxiety agents, sedatives.	• To decrease the patient's anxiety and fear and relieve pain or discomfort
• Encourage the patient and family to take advantage of counseling services and support groups, as appropriate.	• To develop effective coping skills

NURSING DIAGNOSES: ANXIETY *(CONTINUED)*

OUTCOME:	EVALUATION CRITERIA:
• The patient will appear calm and relaxed.	• Physical signs of distress, such as agitation, restlessness, and elevated respiratory rate are decreased or absent.
	• Confidence and relaxation are increased.

NURSING DIAGNOSIS: KNOWLEDGE DEFICIT

RELATED TO:
- *Patient's disorder, treatment plans, diagnostic tests, and procedures*

Nursing Interventions	Rationales
• Explain, using appropriate language, the patient's disorder.	• To increase awareness of the disorder
• Encourage the patient, family members, and other caregivers to ask questions.	• To reinforce their understanding of the patient's disorder and treatment procedures
• Teach the patient necessary self-care routines, as required.	• To promote the feeling of control over the situation
• Explain prescribed medications and their adverse effects, including danger signs that the patient should report to the health care provider.	• To increase understanding of the therapeutic measures
• Describe the danger signs and symptoms that the patient should report to the health care provider, such as difficulty in breathing, especially when lying down or with exertion.	• To increase understanding of the patient's disorder and prevent a respiratory emergency

COLLABORATIVE MANAGEMENT

Interventions	Rationales
• Confer with physicians and other health care providers to identify other situations the patient may experience in the course of treatment.	• To anticipate the patient's need for information and to provide for it before the patient finds himself or herself in an anxiety-producing situation

OUTCOME:	EVALUATION CRITERIA:
• The patient will demonstrate increased understanding of his or her disorder.	• The patient describes the disorder, treatment plans, prescribed medications and adverse effects, and danger signs and symptoms.

NURSING DIAGNOSIS: PAIN

RELATED TO:

- *Injury or trauma, iatrogenic devices needed to ensure respiration and ventilation, or surgical procedures required by the patient's disorder*

Nursing Interventions	Rationales
• Assess the patient's level of discomfort, using a pain scale from 0 to 10.	• To help determine measures to take to adequately combat the pain
• Monitor vital signs for indications of increased pain, such as rapid heart rate and elevated blood pressure.	• To assess for objective signs of worsening pain
• Address the patient's previous experiences with pain and how the patient coped with them.	• To encourage the use of previously successful coping mechanisms for controlling pain
• Teach the patient nonpharmacologic methods for controlling pain, such as meditation, guided imagery, and therapeutic touch.	• To relieve pain

NURSING DIAGNOSIS: PAIN *(CONTINUED)*

Nursing Interventions *(Continued)*	Rationales *(Continued)*
• Teach the patient about the pharmacologic interventions prescribed for him or her.	• To ensure that the patient knows when to ask for medication to prevent pain from becoming intolerable

COLLABORATIVE MANAGEMENT

Interventions	Rationales
• Consult with the pain management specialist about the best modes for treating the patient's pain (for example, when should pain be treated with medication and when should nonpharmacologic pain control methods be used).	• To provide better methods for controlling the pain and discomfort
• Administer medications, as ordered: analgesics.	• To relieve pain

NURSE ALERT:
Sometimes patients are reluctant to give accurate reports of pain, causing health care providers to underestimate the dosage to prescribe or dispense.

OUTCOME:	EVALUATION CRITERIA:
• The patient will have minimal or no pain.	• Pain or discomfort is reported to be decreased or absent.
	• The pain scale rating is 4 or less.

NURSING DIAGNOSIS: HIGH RISK FOR INFECTION

RELATED TO:

- *Trauma or injury or to iatrogenic devices needed to ensure adequate lung expansion*

Nursing Interventions	Rationales
• Monitor the patient for signs of increasing infection, including evaluation of sputum, if appropriate.	• To prevent infection from occurring or worsening
• Monitor the chest tube insertion site for redness, swelling, and tenderness.	• To prevent infection from occurring or worsening
• If the patient is intubated, institute an appropriate hygiene regimen and good pulmonary toilet, including chest physiotherapy and aseptic suctioning techniques.	• To decrease the likelihood of infection
• Encourage the patient to clear secretions from the respiratory passageways and, if needed, suction the secretions. If the patient is not intubated, use deep breathing, cough, and incentive spirometry.	• To reduce the accumulation of secretions, which can lead to infection

COLLABORATIVE MANAGEMENT

Interventions	Rationales
• Administer medications, as ordered: antibiotics.	• To reduce and resolve infection

OUTCOME:

- The patient will remain free of infection, and the chest tube insertion site, if present, will show no signs of infection.

EVALUATION CRITERIA:

- Vital signs and white blood cell count are normal. Pleural fluid cultures are negative.
- Surgical incision or injury, if present, shows no signs of swelling or redness.

Patient Teaching

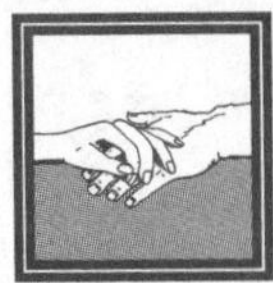

Patient teaching in respiratory emergency situations initially centers around the patient's condition and prognosis. Teaching may be directed toward the patient, if his or her condition permits, or toward the patient's family or other caregivers. In cases of injury such as this, teaching about preventive measures is usually not appropriate. This is especially true if the patient is a child. Note that you may need to repeat information or answer questions repeatedly because the ability to concentrate on new and complicated information is commonly compromised during an emergency.

Once the patient has been stabilized, educate the patient and family about treatment plans, monitoring, and diagnostic procedures and tests.

When the patient is ready for discharge, instruct the patient in self-care routines, preventive measures, and the proper use of prescribed medications. Reinforce information about danger signs that should be reported to the health care provider and any special dietary or activity restrictions.

Documentation

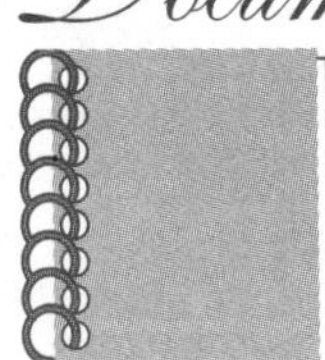

- Ongoing assessment should include the following:
  - Vital signs, especially respiratory rate, effort, and pattern
  - Arterial blood gas analysis
  - Radiography
  - Pulse oximetry
  - Daily weight
- Patient compliance with care regimen
- Patient response to prescribed medications and other therapeutic measures

Chapter 16. Respiratory Failure

▽ ▽ ▽ ▽ ▽ ▽ ▽

Introduction

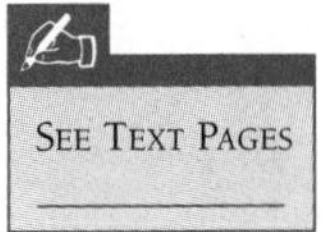

Respiratory failure can result from many conditions, such as injury or trauma, aggravation of chronic conditions, iatrogenic measures, and cardiac complications. There are two forms of respiratory failure: type I, or hypoxemic failure, and type II, or hypercapnic or hypoventilatory failure.

NURSING DIAGNOSES: IMPAIRED GAS EXCHANGE / INEFFECTIVE BREATHING PATTERN

RELATED TO:

- *Respiratory emergency, increased respiratory rate with potential for respiratory fatigue and impending failure*

Nursing Interventions	Rationales
• Observe the patient's chest expansion, tracheal alignment, vital signs, respiratory status (rate effort and regularity), arterial blood gas values, pulse oximetry, and chest radiographs closely. Auscultate breath sounds frequently (every 15 minutes). Evaluate neurologic status closely for confusion or anxiety, which may indicate impending respiratory failure.	• To detect evidence of impending respiratory failure
• Assist the patient to maintain a comfortable position for maximum respiratory benefit, usually high Fowler's position.	• To ease respiration and facilitate diaphragmatic excursion

COLLABORATIVE MANAGEMENT

Interventions	Rationales
• Administer oxygen therapy, as ordered.	• To decrease tissue hypoxia

NURSING DIAGNOSES: IMPAIRED GAS EXCHANGE *(CONTINUED)*

COLLABORATIVE MANAGEMENT *(CONTINUED)*

Interventions *(Continued)*	Rationales *(Continued)*
• Monitor arterial blood gas values and pulse oximetry.	• To detect signs of respiratory failure
• Prepare the patient for intubation and mechanical ventilation.	• To support and maintain patient's respiratory efforts

NURSE ALERT:
Using FiO_2 at levels greater than 60% for an extended period of time (2 to 5 days) puts the patient at risk for oxygen toxicity.

Interventions	Rationales
• Administer medications as ordered: bronchodilators.	• To aid respiratory effort
• If the patient is intubated, suction the airway as needed. Use sterile saline instillations to clear the secretions, if required.	• To ensure adequate respiration and ease the clearing of secretions

OUTCOME:

- The patient will be able to sustain spontaneous ventilation with an easy, regular pattern. Adequate ventilation will occur.

EVALUATION CRITERIA:

- Breathing is relaxed and easy.
- Vital signs are within normal limits.
- Arterial blood gas values are normal.
- There is no evidence of cyanosis.

NURSING DIAGNOSES: ANXIETY
FEAR

RELATED TO:

- *Uncertain outcome of the disorder, dyspnea and other respiratory difficulties, pain, and lack of information about the disorder, treatment plans, diagnostics tests, and procedures*

Nursing Interventions	Rationales
• Explain the disorder to the patient and family members or other caregivers, using appropriate language.	• To ease unfamiliarity and discomfort
• Monitor the patient for signs of increasing distress.	• To prevent levels of anxiety and fear from becoming an additional burden on the patient's condition
• Maintain a calm, relaxed demeanor, and reassure the patient that his or her condition is monitored at all times.	• To prevent additional anxiety concerning the staff's presence and attitude
• Encourage the patient to share his or her concerns, and respond to each as appropriate.	• To maintain open lines of communication
• Promote a quiet environment by reducing external stimulation.	• To limit the drain on the patient's resources —mental, emotional, and physical
• Plan for care activities at times when the patient is feeling best able to handle the stress.	• To avoid unduly stressing the patient

COLLABORATIVE MANAGEMENT

Interventions	Rationales
• Administer medications as ordered: analgesics, antianxiety agents, sedatives.	• To decrease the patient's anxiety and fear and relieve pain or discomfort
• Encourage the patient and family to take advantage of counseling services and support groups, as appropriate.	• To develop effective coping skills

NURSING DIAGNOSES: ANXIETY *(CONTINUED)*

OUTCOME:

- The patient will appear calm and relaxed.

EVALUATION CRITERIA:

- Physical signs of distress, such as agitation, restlessness, and elevated respiratory rate are decreased or absent.
- Confidence and relaxation are increased.

NURSING DIAGNOSIS: KNOWLEDGE DEFICIT

RELATED TO:

- *Patient's disorder, treatment plans, diagnostic tests, and procedures*

Nursing Interventions	Rationales
• Explain, using appropriate language, the patient's disorder.	• To increase awareness of the disorder
• Encourage the patient, family members, and other caregivers to ask questions.	• To reinforce their understanding of the patient's disorder and treatment procedures
• Teach the patient necessary self-care routines, as required.	• To promote the feeling of control over the situation

COLLABORATIVE MANAGEMENT

Interventions	Rationales
• Confer with physicians and other health care providers to identify other situations the patient may experience in the course of treatment.	• To anticipate the patient's need for information and to provide for it before the patient finds himself or herself in an anxiety-producing situation

OUTCOME:

- The patient will demonstrate increased understanding of his or her disorder.

EVALUATION CRITERIA:

- The patient describes the disorder, treatment plans, prescribed medications and adverse effects, and danger signs and symptoms.

NURSING DIAGNOSIS: HIGH RISK FOR INFECTION

RELATED TO:

- *Trauma or injury or to iatrogenic devices needed to ensure adequate lung expansion, mechanical ventilation*

Nursing Interventions	Rationales
• Monitor the patient for signs of increasing infection, including evaluation of sputum, if appropriate.	• To prevent infection from occurring or worsening
• Monitor the chest tube insertion site for redness, swelling, and tenderness.	• To prevent infection from occurring or worsening
• If the patient is intubated, institute an appropriate hygiene regimen and good pulmonary toilet, including chest physiotherapy and aseptic suctioning techniques.	• To decrease the likelihood of infection
• Encourage the patient to clear secretions from the respiratory passageways and, if needed, suction the secretions. If the patient is not intubated, use deep breathing, cough, and incentive spirometry.	• To reduce the accumulation of secretions, which can lead to infection

COLLABORATIVE MANAGEMENT

Interventions	Rationales
• Administer medications, as ordered: antibiotics.	• To reduce and resolve infection

OUTCOME:	EVALUATION CRITERIA:
• The patient will remain free of infection, and the chest tube insertion site, if present, will show no signs of infection.	• Vital signs and white blood cell count are normal. Pleural fluid cultures are negative. • Surgical incision or injury, if present, shows no signs of swelling or redness.

NURSING DIAGNOSIS: INABILITY TO SUSTAIN SPONTANEOUS VENTILATION

RELATED TO:

- *Neurologic causes, infectious processes, and pulmonary complications*

Nursing Interventions	Rationales
• Monitor the patient's vital signs carefully and frequently, especially respiratory status and arterial blood gas values.	• To identify signs of impending respiratory failure
• Assess the patient's level of consciousness.	• To detect signs of agitation, restlessness, or confusion, which may indicate worsening of the patient's condition
• Assist the patient to maintain a comfortable position.	• To facilitate respiratory excursion

COLLABORATIVE MANAGEMENT

Interventions	Rationales
• Administer oxygen, as ordered.	• To ensure adequate oxygenation

OUTCOME:

- The patient will be able to maintain spontaneous ventilation.

EVALUATION CRITERIA:

- Vital signs are normal.
- Respiratory status is normal.
- Arterial blood gas values are within normal ranges.

Patient Teaching

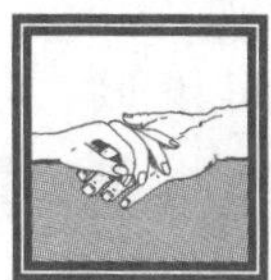

Patient teaching in respiratory emergency situations initially centers around the patient's condition and prognosis. Teaching may be directed toward the patient, if his or her condition permits, or toward the patient's family or other caregivers.

Once the patient has been stabilized, educate the patient and family about treatment plans, monitoring, and diagnostic procedures and tests.

When the patient is ready for discharge, instruct the patient in self-care routines, preventive measures, and the proper use of prescribed medications. Reinforce information about danger signs that should be reported to the health care provider and any special dietary or activity restrictions.

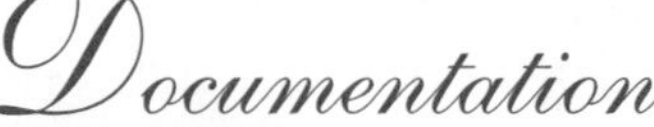

- Ongoing assessment should include the following:
  - Vital signs, especially respiratory rate, effort, and pattern
  - Arterial blood gas analysis
  - Radiography
  - Pulse oximetry
  - Daily weight
- Patient compliance with care regimen
- Patient response to prescribed medications and other therapeutic measures

Chapter 17. Pulmonary Edema and Embolism

Introduction

SEE TEXT PAGES ______

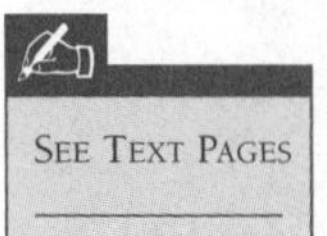

Pulmonary edema is the accumulation of fluid in the alveoli and interstitial spaces of the lung. Pulmonary embolism is the blockage of a main pulmonary artery or one of its branches by a blood clot, air, fat deposit, or other substance.

POTENTIAL SITES OF ORIGIN FOR PULMONARY EMBOLI

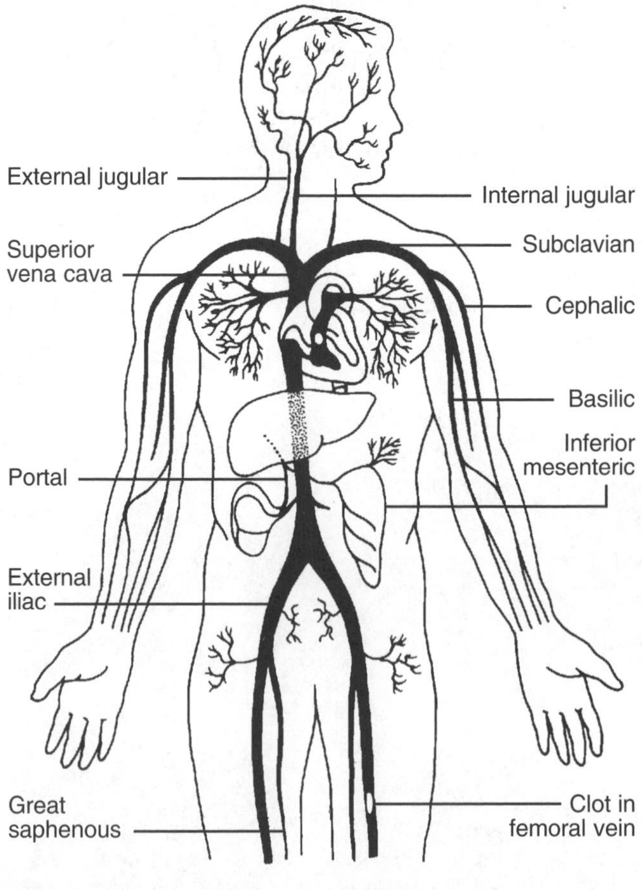

NURSING DIAGNOSES: IMPAIRED GAS EXCHANGE INEFFECTIVE BREATHING PATTERN

RELATED TO:

- *Respiratory emergency and the compromised integrity of pulmonary structures*

Nursing Interventions	Rationales
• Observe the patient's chest expansion, tracheal alignment, vital signs, respiratory status (rate effort and regularity), arterial blood gas values, pulse oximetry, and chest radiographs closely. Auscultate breath sounds frequently (every 15 minutes).	• To monitor baseline functioning and deviations from normal that may indicate complications
• In the patient with suspected pulmonary embolism, assess calf and thigh circumferences, color, and pulses.	• To detect signs of deep vein thrombosis which may lead to pulmonary emboli
• Monitor neck veins for distention in the patient with pulmonary edema.	• To detect signs of pulmonary congestion
• Assist the patient to maintain a comfortable position for maximum respiratory benefit, usually high Fowler's position.	• To ease respiration and facilitate diaphragmatic excursion

NURSE ALERT:
In a patient with pulmonary edema, make sure the feet are dangling to prevent blood engorgement in the lungs. By dangling the feet, venous blood and fluid are prevented from backing up into the lungs.

NURSING DIAGNOSES: IMPAIRED GAS EXCHANGE *(CONTINUED)*

COLLABORATIVE MANAGEMENT

Interventions	Rationales
• Prepare the patient for phlebotomy, if indicated.	• To decrease venous pressure
• Administer oxygen therapy, as ordered.	• To decrease tissue hypoxia
• Monitor arterial blood gas values and pulse oximetry.	• To detect signs of respiratory failure
• Administer medications as ordered: analgesics, anticoagulants (I.V. heparin for pulmonary embolism), bronchodilators, diuretics (for pulmonary edema), sedatives.	• To aid respiratory effort

NURSE ALERT:
When treating a patient with anticoagulants, be sure to closely monitor the patient's coagulation factors (prothrombin time and partial thromboplastin time). When treating a patient with diuretics, be sure to closely monitor the patient's fluid and electrolyte status, especially serum potassium levels.

Interventions	Rationales
• Prepare the patient for diagnostic or therapeutic measures, such as lung perfusion and ventilation scans and pulmonary angiography for pulmonary embolism.	• To ensure ventilation and protect the airway
• If the patient is intubated, suction the airway as needed. Use sterile saline instillations to clear the secretions, if required.	• To ensure adequate respiration and ease the clearing of secretions

NURSING DIAGNOSES: IMPAIRED GAS EXCHANGE *(CONTINUED)*

OUTCOME:

- The patient will be able to sustain spontaneous ventilation with an easy, regular pattern. Adequate ventilation will occur.

EVALUATION CRITERIA:

- Breathing is relaxed and easy.
- Vital signs are within normal limits.
- Arterial blood gas values are normal.
- There is no evidence of cyanosis.

NURSING DIAGNOSES: ANXIETY FEAR

RELATED TO:

- *Uncertain outcome of the disorder, dyspnea and other respiratory difficulties, pain, and lack of information about the disorder, treatment plans, diagnostics tests, and procedures*

Nursing Interventions	Rationales
• Explain the disorder to the patient and family members or other caregivers, using appropriate language.	• To ease unfamiliarity and discomfort
• Monitor the patient for signs of increasing distress.	• To prevent levels of anxiety and fear from becoming an additional burden on the patient's condition
• Maintain a calm, relaxed demeanor, and reassure the patient that his or her condition is monitored at all times.	• To prevent additional anxiety concerning the staff's presence and attitude
• Encourage the patient to share his or her concerns, and respond to each as appropriate.	• To maintain open lines of communication
• Promote a quiet environment by reducing external stimulation.	• To limit the drain on the patient's resources—mental, emotional, and physical

NURSING DIAGNOSES: ANXIETY *(CONTINUED)*

COLLABORATIVE MANAGEMENT

Interventions	Rationales
• Plan for care activities at times when the patient is feeling best able to handle the stress.	• To avoid unduly stressing the patient
• Administer medications as ordered: analgesics, antianxiety agents, sedatives.	• To decrease the patient's anxiety and fear and relieve pain or discomfort
• Encourage the patient and family to take advantage of counseling services and support groups, as appropriate.	• To develop effective coping skills

OUTCOME:	EVALUATION CRITERIA:
• The patient will appear calm and relaxed.	• Physical signs of distress, such as agitation, restlessness, and elevated respiratory rate are decreased or absent. • Confidence and relaxation are increased.

NURSING DIAGNOSIS: KNOWLEDGE DEFICIT

RELATED TO:

- *Patient's disorder, treatment plans, diagnostic tests, and procedures*

Nursing Interventions	Rationales
• Explain, using appropriate language, the patient's disorder.	• To increase awareness of the disorder
• Encourage the patient, family members, and other caregivers to ask questions.	• To reinforce their understanding of the patient's disorder and treatment procedures
• Teach the patient necessary self-care routines, as required.	• To promote the feeling of control over the situation

Nursing Interventions *(Continued)*

- Explain prescribed medications and their adverse effects, including danger signs that the patient should report to the health care provider.

Rationales *(Continued)*

- To increase understanding of the therapeutic measures

NURSE ALERT:
Inform a patient receiving anticoagulant therapy for pulmonary embolism that he or she can prevent bleeding by using an electric razors and a soft toothbrush. Review signs of venous stasis with the patient, and explain ways to avoid embolism formation, such as wearing loose-fitting clothes and not sitting in one position too long.

Teach the patient receiving diuretic therapy for pulmonary edema about potential adverse effects, activity and dietary limitations, and danger signs of pulmonary congestion.

- Describe the danger signs and symptoms that the patient should report to the health care provider, such as difficulty in breathing, especially when lying down or with exertion.

- To increase understanding of the patient's disorder and prevent a respiratory emergency

COLLABORATIVE MANAGEMENT

Interventions

- Confer with physicians and other health care providers to identify other situations the patient may experience in the course of treatment.

Rationales

- To anticipate the patient's need for information and to provide for it before the patient finds himself or herself in an anxiety-producing situation

NURSING DIAGNOSIS: KNOWLEDGE DEFICIT *(CONTINUED)*

OUTCOME:	EVALUATION CRITERIA:
• The patient will demonstrate increased understanding of his or her disorder.	• The patient describes the disorder, treatment plans, prescribed medications and adverse effects, and danger signs and symptoms.

NURSING DIAGNOSIS: PAIN

RELATED TO:

- *Pulmonary embolism, injury or trauma, iatrogenic devices needed to ensure respiration and ventilation, or surgical procedures required by the patient's disorder*

Nursing Interventions	Rationales
• Assess the patient's level of discomfort, using a pain scale from 0 to 10.	• To help determine measures to take to adequately combat the pain
• Monitor vital signs for indications of increased pain, such as rapid heart rate and elevated blood pressure.	• To assess for objective signs of worsening pain
• Address the patient's previous experiences with pain and how the patient coped with them.	• To encourage the use of previously successful coping mechanisms for controlling pain
• Teach the patient nonpharmacologic methods for controlling pain, such as meditation, guided imagery, and therapeutic touch.	• To relieve pain
• Teach patient about the pharmacologic interventions prescribed for him or her.	• To ensure that the patient knows when to ask for medication to prevent pain from becoming intolerable

COLLABORATIVE MANAGEMENT

Interventions	Rationales
• Consult with the pain management specialist about the best modes for treating the patient's pain (for example, when should pain be treated with medication and when should nonpharmacologic pain control methods be used).	• To provide better methods for controlling the pain and discomfort
• Administer medications, as ordered: analgesics.	• To relieve pain

NURSE ALERT:
Sometimes patients are reluctant to give accurate reports of pain, causing health care providers to underestimate the dosage to prescribe or dispense.

OUTCOME:	EVALUATION CRITERIA:
• The patient will have minimal or no pain.	• Pain or discomfort is reported to be decreased or absent. • The pain scale rating is 4 or less.

NURSING DIAGNOSIS: HIGH RISK FOR INFECTION

RELATED TO:
- *Trauma or injury or to iatrogenic devices needed to ensure adequate lung expansion*

Nursing Interventions	Rationales
• Monitor the patient for signs of increasing infection, including evaluation of sputum, if appropriate.	• To prevent infection from occurring or worsening

NURSING DIAGNOSIS: HIGH RISK FOR INFECTION *(CONTINUED)*

Nursing Interventions *(Continued)*	Rationales *(Continued)*
• If the patient is intubated, institute an appropriate hygiene regimen and good pulmonary toilet, including aseptic suctioning techniques.	• To decrease the likelihood of infection
• Encourage the patient to clear secretions from the respiratory passageways and, if needed, suction the secretions. If the patient is not intubated, use deep breathing, cough, and incentive spirometry.	• To reduce the accumulation of secretions, which can lead to infection

COLLABORATIVE MANAGEMENT

Interventions	Rationales
• Administer medications, as ordered: antibiotics.	• To reduce and resolve infection

OUTCOME:	EVALUATION CRITERIA:
• The patient will remain free of infection, and the chest tube insertion site, if present, will show no signs of infection.	• Vital signs and white blood cell count are normal. Pleural fluid cultures are negative. • Surgical incision or injury, if present, shows no signs of swelling or redness.

NURSING DIAGNOSIS: DECREASED CARDIAC OUTPUT

RELATED TO:
- *Pulmonary edema*

Nursing Interventions	Rationales
• Monitor the patient for signs of cardiac distress, including decreasing mental status, decreasing blood pressure,	• To anticipate the need for resuscitative measures

Nursing Interventions *(Continued)*	Rationales *(Continued)*
increasing heart rate and rhythm, unequal chest expansion, and tracheal deviation.	
• Assure that emergency resuscitative equipment is readily available for immediate use.	• To promote fast, effective treatment
• Prepare the patient for therapeutic measures, such as chest tube insertion and thoracentesis for pneumothorax or tension pneumothorax.	• To relieve pressure on the heart and great vessels and help restore cardiac output

COLLABORATIVE MANAGEMENT

Interventions	Rationales
• Assist with diagnostic procedures, especially pulmonary artery catheterization and central venous pressure monitoring.	• To provide accurate information for use by the staff, if needed
• Initiate oxygen therapy, as ordered.	• To prevent tissue hypoxia
• Monitor arterial blood gas values and pulse oximetry.	• To identify signs of respiratory failure

OUTCOME:	EVALUATION CRITERIA:
• The patient will maintain adequate cardiac output for his or her age and body surface area.	• Blood pressure is normal. • Pulse rate is strong and regular. • Mental status is clear. • Heartbeat pattern is normal. • Jugular vein is not distended.

Patient Teaching

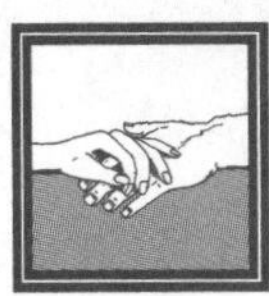

When the patient is ready for discharge, instruct the patient in self-care routines, preventive measures, and the proper use of prescribed medications. Reinforce information about danger signs that should be reported to the health care provider and any special dietary or activity restrictions.

Identify measures the patient should take to avoid the formation of emboli, such as:

- Avoiding extended periods of immobility, especially sitting with crossed legs
- Eliminating the use of hosiery with tight thigh, knee, or ankle bands

Explain the role of smoking in increasing vasoconstriction. Educate the patient about the importance of a low-sodium, low-fat diet.

Documentation

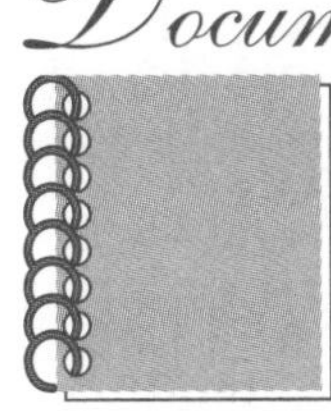

- Ongoing assessment should include the following:
  - Vital signs, especially respiratory rate, effort, and pattern
  - Arterial blood gas analysis
  - Radiography
  - Pulse oximetry
  - Daily weight
- Patient compliance with care regimen
- Patient response to prescribed medications and other therapeutic measures

Chapter 18. Adult Respiratory Distress Syndrome

▽ ▽ ▽ ▽ ▽ ▽ ▽

Introduction

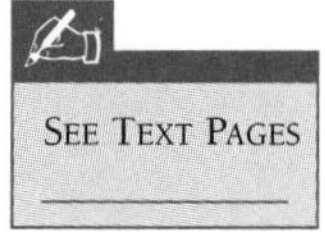

Adult respiratory distress syndrome (ARDS), a type of respiratory failure, can result from many conditions and disorders. It is not known why this syndrome presents identically in all cases, despite the wide variety of causative factors.

NURSE ALERT:
This disorder is also called shock lung, stiff lung, noncardiac pulmonary edema, wet lung, white lung, Da Nang lung, and adult hyaline membrane disease, although the term ARDS is the most widely accepted.

NURSING DIAGNOSES: IMPAIRED GAS EXCHANGE INEFFECTIVE BREATHING PATTERN

RELATED TO:
- *Decreased lung compliance and increased respiratory effort and lung consolidation*

Nursing Interventions	Rationales
• Monitor the patient's respiratory pattern for rate, effort, and regularity. Auscultate for breath sounds, and assess arterial blood gas values and pulse oximetry.	• To prevent further respiratory difficulties and establish a baseline

NURSE ALERT:
Be especially alert for signs of spontaneous pneumothorax, which may be caused by increased airway pressure.

NURSING DIAGNOSES: IMPAIRED GAS EXCHANGE *(CONTINUED)*

Nursing Interventions *(Continued)*	Rationales *(Continued)*
• Maintain the patient in a slight reverse Trendelenburg position.	• To ease respiration by keeping the abdominal contents from resting on the diaphragm and helping to prevent further increases in airway pressure
• If the patient has been intubated and placed on mechanical ventilation, perform suction, as needed. Use sterile saline instillations to clear the secretions, if required.	• To clear secretions

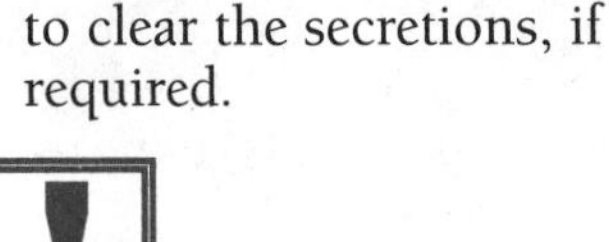

NURSE ALERT:
Be careful not to disconnect the patient from the ventilator if pressure control ventilation or high positive-end expiratory pressure (PEEP) levels are being used because this may cause severe hypoxia.

Nursing Interventions *(Continued)*	Rationales *(Continued)*
• Document peak, pause, and mean airway pressures from the mechanical ventilator.	• To monitor the patient's baseline and assess trends that may indicate a worsening of the patient's condition
• Document the patient's fluid intake and output.	• To prevent fluid overload

COLLABORATIVE MANAGEMENT

Interventions	Rationales
• Use the appropriate means of mechanical ventilation, either volume-cycled mode or pressure-control mode, as ordered.	• To ensure adequate ventilation at the alveolar level
• Administer sedatives, as ordered, especially before suctioning.	• To decrease oxygen demand and prevent further increases in airway pressure

COLLABORATIVE MANAGEMENT *(CONTINUED)*

Interventions *(Continued)*	Rationales *(Continued)*
• Assist with the placement of a pulmonary artery (PA) catheter.	• To monitor left-sided heart functioning and fluid volume status
• Administer oxygen therapy, as ordered. Oxygen therapy is usually required until fraction of inspired oxygen levels reach a danger point (greater than 60% for several days) or the patient is placed on mechanical ventilation.	• To ease respiration and facilitate ventilation
• Monitor arterial blood gas and pulse oximetry values closely.	• To detect early signs of respiratory failure
• Assist with intubation procedures, if required.	• To ensure respiration
• Working with the physician and respiratory therapists, develop a plan for mechanical ventilation, including ventilation mode, inspiratory and expiratory ratios, PEEP levels, and permissible levels of hypercapnia.	• To promote adequate respiration using lower airway pressures at the cost of higher carbon dioxide levels. Lower airway pressure results in lower alveolar pressures, which may allow the damaged lung tissue time to heal.

NURSE ALERT:
Possible alternative ventilation methods include high-frequency jet ventilation and extracorporeal membrane oxygenation in extreme cases.

Interventions	Rationales
• Administer medications, as ordered: neuromuscular blockers, sedatives.	• To decrease patient activity requiring increased respiratory efforts

NURSING DIAGNOSES: IMPAIRED GAS EXCHANGE *(CONTINUED)*

OUTCOME:

- The patient will be able to sustain spontaneous ventilation with an easy, regular pattern and adequate gas exchange.

EVALUATION CRITERIA:

- Breathing is relaxed and easy.
- Vital signs are within normal limits.
- Arterial blood gas values are normal.
- There is no evidence of cyanosis.
- Pulse oximetry levels are acceptable (usually greater than 90%).

NURSING DIAGNOSIS: DECREASED CARDIAC OUTPUT

RELATED TO:

- *Increased intrathoracic pressures secondary to positive-pressure ventilation and high PEEP, which increase intrathoracic pressures and decrease venous return, causing a decrease in cardiac output*

Nursing Interventions	Rationales
• Monitor the patient for signs of cardiac distress, including decreasing mental status, decreasing blood pressure, and increasing heart rate and rhythm.	• To anticipate the need for resuscitative measures and corrective interventions
• Monitor and document PA catheter readings, and note the effect of any medications ordered.	• To measure the effectiveness of treatment
• Monitor urine output.	• To determine the adequacy of tissue perfusion (renal) and prevent renal failure

COLLABORATIVE MANAGEMENT

Interventions	Rationales
• Assist with diagnostic procedures, such as PA catheter insertion and central venous pressure monitoring.	• To provide accurate information for use by the staff
• Titrate oxygen therapy, as ordered.	• To increase the effectiveness of ventilation
• Administer and titrate medications, as ordered: diuretics, ionotropes, I.V. fluids, vasopressors.	• To promote effective perfusion

OUTCOME:

- The patient will maintain adequate cardiac output for his or her age and body surface area.

EVALUATION CRITERIA:

- Blood pressure is normal.
- Pulse rate is strong and regular.
- Mental status is clear.
- Heartbeat pattern is normal.
- Jugular veins are not distended.

NURSING DIAGNOSES: ANXIETY
FEAR
INEFFECTIVE FAMILY COPING
INEFFECTIVE INDIVIDUAL COPING

RELATED TO:

- *Uncertain outcome of the disorder, respiratory difficulties, and lack of information about the disorder, treatment plans, diagnostics tests, and procedures*

Nursing Interventions	Rationales
• Explain the disorder to the patient, family members, or other caregivers, using appropriate language.	• To ease unfamiliarity and discomfort

NURSING DIAGNOSES: ANXIETY *(CONTINUED)*

Nursing Interventions *(Continued)*	Rationales *(Continued)*
• Monitor the patient for signs of increasing distress.	• To prevent levels of anxiety and fear from becoming an additional burden on the patient's condition
• Maintain a calm, relaxed demeanor, and reassure the patient that his or her condition is monitored at all times.	• To prevent additional anxiety concerning the staff's presence and attitude
• Encourage the patient to share his or her concerns, and respond to each as appropriate.	• To maintain open lines of communication
• Promote a quiet environment by reducing external stimulation.	• To limit the drain on patient's resources—mental, emotional, and physical
• Plan for care activities at times when the patient is feeling best able to handle the stress.	• To avoid unduly stressing the patient

COLLABORATIVE MANAGEMENT

Interventions	Rationales
• Administer medications, as ordered: sedatives.	• To decrease anxiety and fear
• Encourage the patient and family members to take advantage of counseling services and support groups, as appropriate.	• To develop effective coping skills

OUTCOME:	EVALUATION CRITERIA:
• The patient will appear calm and relaxed.	• Physical signs of distress, such as agitation, restlessness, and elevated respiratory rate are decreased or absent.
• The patient and family will demonstrate healthy coping mechanisms.	• Confidence and relaxation are increased.

Patient Teaching

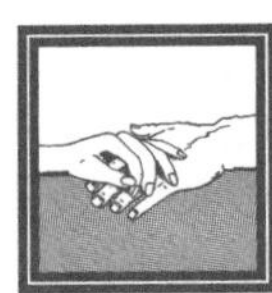

Patient teaching for the patient with ARDS initially centers around the patient's condition and prognosis. Teaching may be directed toward the patient, if the patient's condition permits, or toward the patient's family or other caregivers.

Explain that the patient will, at some point, be intubated and placed on mechanical ventilation. When this occurs, the goals for care are to ensure the patency of the endotracheal tube and to continually evaluate the efficacy of the mechanical ventilation efforts.

Once the patient has been stabilized, educate the patient and family about treatment plans, monitoring, and diagnostic procedures and tests, if appropriate.

If it is apparent that the patient will not recover, direct your efforts toward helping the family and other caregivers cope with the situation.

If the patient will be discharged, instruct the patient in self-care routines and preventive measures. Reinforce information about danger signs that should be reported to the health care provider.

Documentation

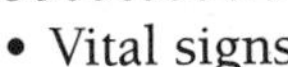

- Vital signs
- Patient response to therapy
- Fluid intake and output
- Left-sided heart function (PA catheter readings)
- Fluid volume status
- Peak, mean, and pause airway pressures

Nursing Research

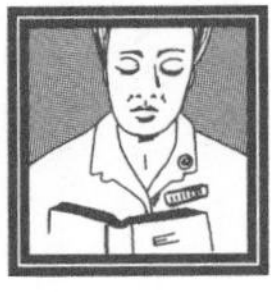

Extracorporeal membrane oxygenation is a new method of managing the ventilation requirements of a patient with ARDS. Blood is pumped into external "lungs," where carbon dioxide is removed and oxygen is added. Blood is processed and then returned to the body, reducing the lungs' workload. This reduction in effort may allow the lungs to heal.

Dirkes, S. "Acute Respiratory Failure and ECMO." *Critical Care Nurse* 12 (October 1992): 39–46.

Surfactant replacement therapy may help to improve lung function and increase the effectiveness of gas exchange. This therapy has not undergone sufficient trial to determine its efficacy.

Sinski, A. "Surfactant Replacement in Adults and Children with ARDS—An Effective Therapy?" *Critical Care Nurse* 14 (December 1994): 54–58.

Suggested Readings

Chillcott, S., and P. S. Sheridan. "Treating ARDS with $ECCO_2$." *Critical Care Nurse* 15, no. 2 (1995): 50–56.

Robertson, O. "Penetrating Chest Trauma: Resolving Life-Threatening Complications." *Nursing95* 25, no. 3 (1995): 33.

Smith, N., J. Fallentine, and S. Kessel. "Underwater Chest Drainage: Bringing the Facts to the Surface." *Nursing95* 25, no. 2 (1995): 60–63.

Smith, N., J. Fallentine, S. Kessel, and M. Maloney. "Instilling the Facts About Autotransfusion." *Nursing95* 25, no. 3 (1995): 52–55.

SECTION VII: OTHER RESPIRATORY DISORDERS

Chapter 19: Pleural Infections

Introduction

SEE TEXT PAGES ______

Infections of the pleura can involve the pleural membranes directly or result from lesions that occupy the pleural space. Pleural infections include the following:

- Pleurisy, inflammation of the visceral or parietal pleura caused by various conditions or diseases. Its most common presentation is that of sharp, unilateral pain of abrupt onset.
- Pleural effusion, the collection of fluid in the pleural space. This space normally contains a small amount of serous fluid that serves to keep the parietal and visceral pleuras in constant contact. The movement of blood, transudate, exudate, or chyle into this space occurs when the rate of removal is surpassed by the rate at which material enters the space.
- Pulmonary fibrosis, a general term for a collection of diseases whose effect on the lungs is that of restriction. Generally, the lung parenchyma stiffens, making respiration difficult.

NURSING DIAGNOSES: IMPAIRED GAS EXCHANGE
INABILITY TO SUSTAIN SPONTANEOUS VENTILATION
INEFFECTIVE AIRWAY CLEARANCE
INEFFECTIVE BREATHING PATTERN

RELATED TO:

- *Pleural infection, chest wall rigidity, and pain, which make respiration difficult*

Nursing Interventions	Rationales
• Monitor respiratory status (for rate, effort, and breath sounds) and vital signs.	• To identify impending respiratory failure

NURSING DIAGNOSES: IMPAIRED GAS EXCHANGE (*CONTINUED*)

Nursing Interventions *(Continued)*	Rationales *(Continued)*
• Elevate the patient's head and back (high Fowler's position), and arrange pillows to support the patient's respiratory efforts.	• To facilitate diaphragmatic excursion, keep the airway open, and alleviate discomfort during breathing
• Encourage the patient to expectorate secretions or perform suction, if needed.	• To clear secretions from the respiratory passageways
• Teach the patient breathing exercises, such as incentive spirometry.	• To open alveolar passages and increase sputum expectoration
• Assist in performing chest physiotherapy, as needed.	• To help mobilize and eliminate lung secretions
• Encourage the patient to drink adequate amounts of fluid (1,500 to 2,000 mL daily).	• To help loosen secretions and compensate for fluid loss from secretion expectoration and elevated temperature
• Use a room humidifier to increase the ambient humidity.	• To assist in liquefying secretions for easier clearing
• Plan patient activities to allow for periods of rest.	• To prevent fatigue and the need for increased respiratory effort
• If the patient is intubated, suction the airway, as needed. Use sterile saline instillations to clear secretions, if required.	• To promote adequate respiration and clear secretions

COLLABORATIVE MANAGEMENT

Interventions	Rationales
• Administer oxygen therapy, as ordered.	• To ensure tissue oxygenation
• Monitor arterial blood gas and pulse oximetry values closely.	• To identify signs of respiratory failure

COLLABORATIVE MANAGEMENT *(CONTINUED)*

Interventions *(Continued)*	Rationales *(Continued)*
• Administer medications, as ordered: antibiotics, antipyretics, bronchodilators, diuretics.	• To resolve respiratory congestion, control fever, and reduce or prevent infection
• Working with respiratory and physical therapists, develop a plan for physical therapy activities (for example, percussion, postural drainage, and ambulation).	• To promote adequate respiration while limiting stress and fatigue
• Assist with surgical incision, drainage, and diagnostic procedures, if ordered.	• To maintain a patent airway
• Maintain and monitor chest tube system, if one is used.	• To ensure a patent airway

OUTCOME:

- The patient will be able to breathe easily and effectively, sustain adequate ventilation and maintain arterial blood gas values within normal ranges. Tissue oxygenation will not be compromised.

EVALUATION CRITERIA:

- Respirations are even and bilateral.
- Edema of affected tissues is decreased.
- Pain or discomfort is reported to be decreased.
- Uvula is located at midline.
- Radiographic findings show resolution.
- Vital signs are within normal limits.
- There is no evidence of cyanosis.
- Arterial blood gas values are within normal ranges.
- Breath sounds are clear on auscultation.

NURSING DIAGNOSES: ANXIETY
FEAR

RELATED TO:

- *Uncertain outcome of the disorder, respiratory difficulties, and lack of information about the disorder, treatment plans, diagnostic tests, and procedures*

Nursing Interventions	Rationales
• Explain the disorder to the patient and family members or other caregivers, using appropriate language for the patient's level of understanding.	• To ease unfamiliarity and discomfort and allow the patient some control over the situation
• Monitor the patient for signs of increasing distress.	• To prevent levels of anxiety and fear from becoming an additional burden on the patient's condition
• Maintain a calm, relaxed demeanor, and reassure the patient that his or her condition is monitored at all times.	• To prevent additional anxiety concerning the staff's presence and attitude
• Encourage the patient to share his or her concerns, and respond to each as appropriate.	• To maintain open lines of communication
• Promote a quiet environment by reducing external stimulation.	• To limit the drain on the patient's resources—mental, emotional, and physical
• Plan for care activities at times when the patient is feeling best able to handle the stress.	• To avoid unduly stressing the patient

COLLABORATIVE MANAGEMENT

Interventions	Rationales
• Administer medications, as ordered: sedatives.	• To decrease anxiety and fear
• Encourage the patient and family members to take advantage of counseling services and support groups, as appropriate.	• To develop effective coping skills

NURSING DIAGNOSES: ANXIETY *(CONTINUED)*

OUTCOME:	EVALUATION CRITERIA:
• The patient will appear calm and relaxed.	• Physical signs of distress, such as agitation, restlessness, and elevated respiratory rate are decreased or absent.
	• Confidence and relaxation are increased.

NURSING DIAGNOSIS: KNOWLEDGE DEFICIT

RELATED TO:

- *Patient's disorder, treatment plans, and diagnostic tests and procedures*

Nursing Interventions	Rationales
• Educate the patient about the pathophysiology of the disease, prescribed medications and adverse effects, follow-up care requirements, and danger signs that should be reported to the health care provider.	• To increase understanding
• Include the patient's family and other caregivers in the educational program.	• To increase the likelihood that the self-care regimen will be followed

COLLABORATIVE MANAGEMENT

Interventions	Rationales
• Refer the patient, family, and other caregivers to the appropriate support agencies.	• To encourage understanding of the disorder
• Collaborate with other health care providers in stressing the importance of the health care regimen.	• To ensure understanding of the importance of the health care regimen

NURSING DIAGNOSIS: KNOWLEDGE DEFICIT *(CONTINUED)*

OUTCOME:

- The patient will demonstrate adequate knowledge about the disorder and self-care routines.

EVALUATION CRITERIA:

- The patient accurately describes the physical effects of the disorder.
- The patient verbalizes an understanding of the use of prescribed medications, their adverse effects, and danger signs.
- The patient complies with follow-up appointments and the self-care regimen.
- The patient seeks health care if conditions indicate the need.

NURSING DIAGNOSIS: PAIN

RELATED TO:

- *Iatrogenic devices needed to ensure respiration and ventilation, surgical procedures required by the patient's disorder or pleural pain associated with an infectious process*

Nursing Interventions	Rationales
• Assess the patient's level of discomfort, using a pain scale from 0 to 10.	• To help determine measures to take to adequately combat pain
• Monitor vital signs for indications of increased pain, such as rapid heart rate and elevated blood pressure.	• To assess for objective signs of worsening pain
• Address the patient's previous experiences with pain and how the patient coped with them.	• To encourage use of previously successful coping mechanisms for controlling pain
• Teach the patient nonpharmacologic methods for controlling pain, such as meditation, guided imagery, and therapeutic touch.	• To relieve pain

Nursing Interventions *(Continued)*	Rationales *(Continued)*
• Teach the patient about the pharmacologic interventions prescribed for him or her.	• To ensure that the patient knows when to ask for medication to prevent pain from becoming intolerable

COLLABORATIVE MANAGEMENT

Interventions	Rationales
• Consult the pain management specialist about the best modes for treating the patient's pain (for example, when should pain be treated with medication or when should nonpharmacologic pain control methods be used).	• To provide better methods for controlling pain and discomfort
• Administer medications, as ordered: analgesics, antibiotics, anti-inflammatory agents.	• To relieve pain and resolve infection

NURSE ALERT:
Sometimes patients are reluctant to give accurate reports of pain, causing health care providers to underestimate the dosage to prescribe or dispense.

Interventions	Rationales
• Assist with surgical procedures, if ordered.	• To relieve pain

NURSE ALERT:
Be especially careful to ensure correct functioning of the chest tube system.

NURSING DIAGNOSIS: PAIN *(CONTINUED)*

OUTCOME:

- The patient will have minimal or no pain.

EVALUATION CRITERIA:

- Pain is reported to be decreased or absent.
- The pain scale rating is 4 or less.

Patient Teaching

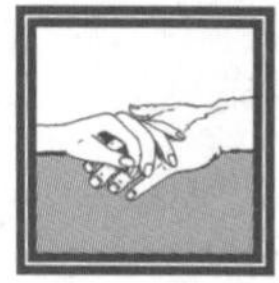

Instruct the patient about his or her disorder, its likely causes if they are known, and what diagnostic and treatment procedures are available.

Identify measures the patient can take to gain control over his or her disorder, such as restricting exposure to smoke, planning activities to take advantage of periods of relative strength, and limiting stress.

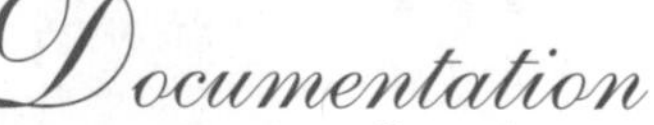

Documentation

- Ongoing assessment should include the following:
  - Vital signs, especially respiratory rate, effort, and pattern and breath sounds
  - Laboratory test results, arterial blood gas analysis, radiographic findings, and pleural fluid cultures
- Patient compliance with self-care regimen
- Patient response to prescribed medication and other therapeutic measures
- If the patient is intubated, amount and character of drainage and the condition of the chest tube insertion site

INDEX

A

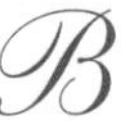

D

F

H

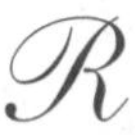

S

T

U

W

ORDER OTHER TITLES IN THIS SERIES!

INSTANT NURSING ASSESSMENT:

▲ Cardiovascular	0-8273-7102-0
▲ Respiratory	0-8273-7099-7
▲ Neurologic	0-8273-7103-9
▲ Women's Health	0-8273-7100-4
▲ Gerontologic	0-8273-7101-2
▲ Mental Health	0-8273-7104-7
▲ Pediatric	0-8273-7098-9

RAPID NURSING INTERVENTIONS

▲ Cardiovascular	0-8273-7105-5
▲ Respiratory	0-8273-7095-4
▲ Neurologic	0-8273-7093-8
▲ Women's Health	0-8273-7092-X
▲ Gerontologic	0-8273-7094-6
▲ Mental Health	0-8273-7096-2
▲ Pediatric	0-8273-7097-0

(cut here)

EXPERIENCE AT YOUR FINGERTIPS!

QTY.	TITLE / ISBN	PRICE	TOTAL
		19.95	
		19.95	
		19.95	
		19.95	
		19.95	
		19.95	
		SUBTOTAL	
		STATE OR LOCAL TAXES	
		TOTAL	

Payment Information

☐ A Check is Enclosed

☐ Charge my ☐ VISA ☐ Mastercard CARD #__________

MAIL OR FAX COMPLETED FORM TO:

Delmar Publishers • P.O. Box 15015 • Albany, NY 12212-5015

NAME________________

SCHOOL/INSTITUTION ________________

STREET ADDRESS________________

CITY/STATE/ZIP ________________

HOME PHONE________________

OFFICE PHONE________________

IN A HURRY TO ORDER? FAX: 1-518-464-0301
OR CALL TOLL-FREE 1-800-347-7707

Delmar's

Rapid Nursing Intervention Series

Respiratory

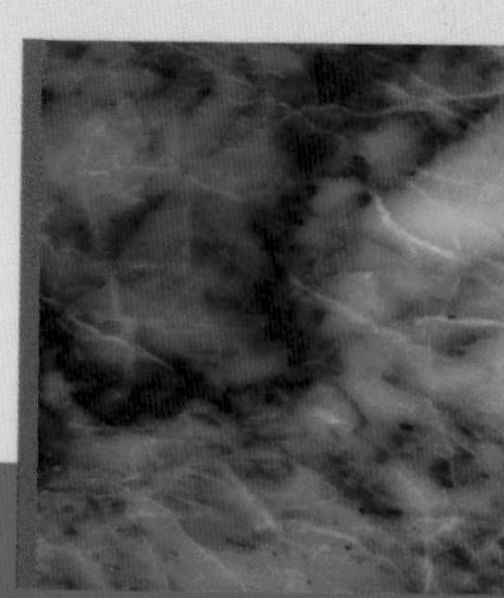

A quick source for appropriate step-by-step nursing actions to help provide quality care and meet the "rapid" challenges of today's nursing profession.

Features

- Nursing diagnoses charts that include interventions and rationales
- Emphasis on collaborative management
- Appropriate outcomes and evaluation criteria
- Patient teaching information stressing preventive/health promotion techniques

ISBN 0-8273-7095-4
90000
9 780827 370951

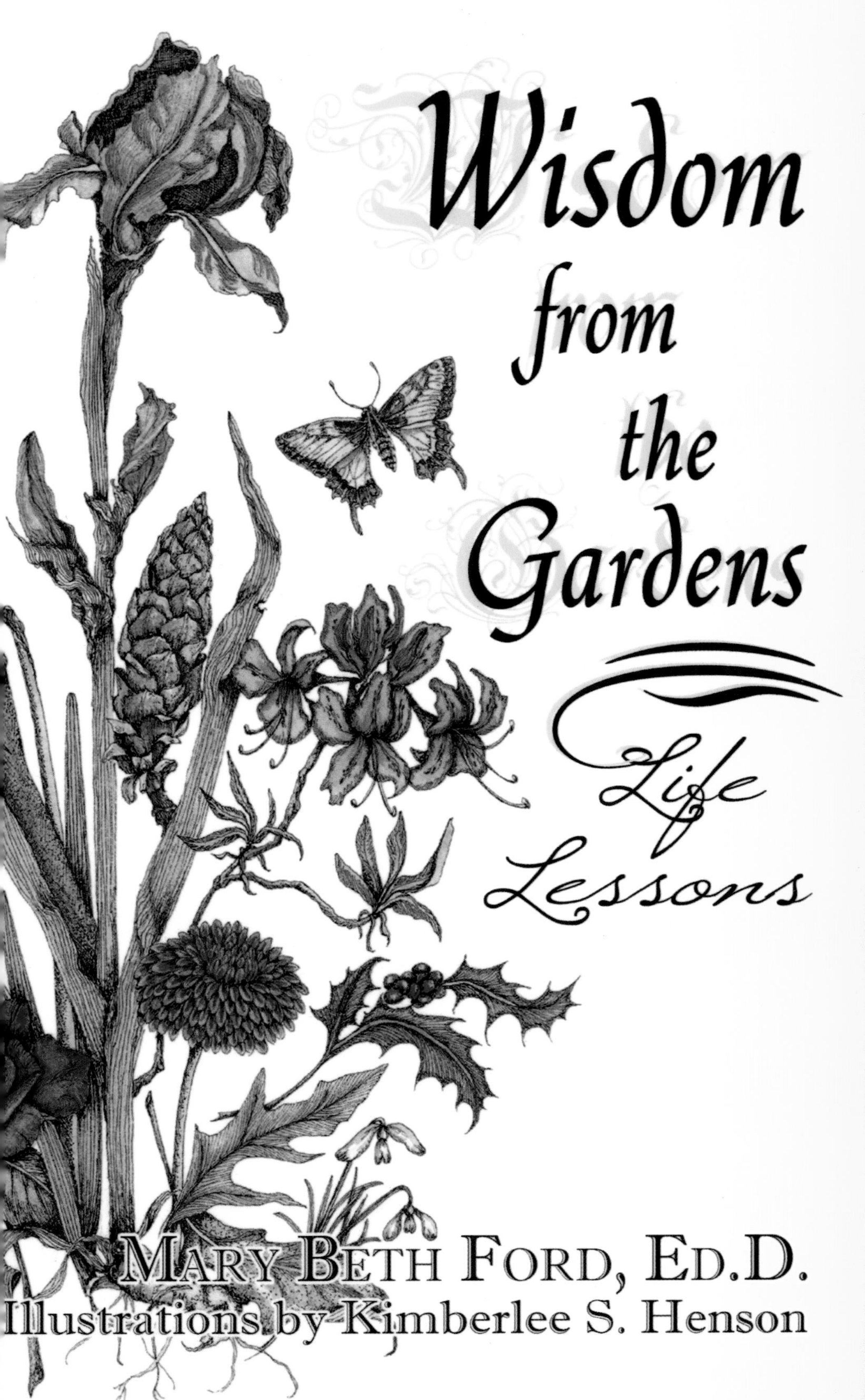
Wisdom
from
the
Gardens
Life
Lessons
Mary Beth Ford, Ed.D.
Illustrations by Kimberlee S. Henson